"Any athlete looking to improve your speed, energy, and mental focus, this book is a must-read!"

    Dave Stockton Jr., PGA Champions Tour

"Pro athlete or not, you will benefit from Justin's book. His protocols and strategies can help anyone wanting to have more success in developing speed."

    Dr. Kevin Priestley, Priestley Chiropractic

"Your strategies for handling energy, speed, and performance are creative, effective, and fun!"

    Lee Holden, Qi Gong Master

"Justin Frandson has written a must-read for anyone considering elevating their game. Read his book and learn from one of the best."

    Dr. Barre Paul Lando, Alfavedic.com

"Having the honor and privilege of knowing and working with Justin for close to twenty years, the information he presents in this book is what he's learned on his own journey and integrated into his own practice. Presented in this book is invaluable knowledge to assist pro athletes, weekend warriors, anyone who wants to feel and look vibrant, dynamic, and be flexible with integrity!

It's an easy read to understand and apply for all ages. Who doesn't want to be their own best healer? We're all here to feel good and have fun on the journey, this book will show you how! Why not!"

    Love *Light
    Kent "Cosmic mechanic"
    Creator/teacher "Wingwork technique"

"Any pro, college, or high school athlete will benefit from Justin's book. His protocols and strategies can help anyone wanting to have more success in adding a new dimension to their game and in helping each individual to become the best he/she can be."

    Steve Conti
    Corona Del Mar High/Middle School
    Physical Education Teacher
    Surf Team Coach

Copyright © 2021 by Justin Frandson

All rights reserved. No part of this book may be reproduced in any manner without written permission except in the case of brief quotations included in critical articles and reviews. For information, please contact the author.

The health information contained in this book is for educational purposes only and does not constitute medical advice or a guarantee of treatment, outcome, or cure. Please consult with your healthcare provider for specific medical advice.

Printed and Bound in The United States of America

First published in 2021 by Sheridan

ISBN 978-0-578-76891-5

First Edition 2021

Cover Design Copyright © 2021 by Jessica Frandson

Illustrations by Kerri Schuh

Editing by Heather Marsh at Classic Editing | HolisticEditing@gmail.com

Book Design by Lam H. Nguyen | www.apercher.com | info@apercher.com

Book Design V27

ATHLETICISM
WHOLE BODY + WHOLE BRAIN = PERFORMANCE

TAKE YOUR ENERGY, SPEED & COORDINATION TO A NEW DIMENSION

FOR ALL LEVELS | Sports or Activities

WWW.ATHLETICISM.COM

ATHLETICISM Performance Coach | **Justin Frandson**, APC, CPT

Foreword by | **Jason Cabell**, 20-Year Retired Navy SEAL
Hollywood Writer / Director / Producer

CONTENTS.

Foreword.

X. Huge accolades for Justin Frandson and this book by Jason Cabell, 20-Year Retired Navy SEAL, Hollywood Writer, Director, and Producer.

Prologue.

X. Benefits to High Level Performance.

XX. Amateur and Professional Athletes, Weekend Warriors, Doctors, Trainers, Therapists, Parents, Active Enthusiasts, Strength Coaches, and All Industry Practitioners, this book is for you.

XXX. We are all athletes able to improve performance in any chosen activity.

In the Trenches.

X. Brain Typing.

XX. History of the Program With Ernie Grunfeld, GM, Washington Wizards and Coach Scott Brooks.

XXX. The 3 Pillars.

XXXX. No Matter Your Sport, Activity, or Level, You Will Improve.

Background.

X. Improper Food.

XX. Health Challenges.

XXX. Growing Up in So Cal.

XXXX. Stephen Stiteler, L.Ac.
XXXXX. My Legendary Mentor, Dean Brittenham & Scripps Clinic, La Jolla, California.

XXXXXX. Amazing Results Compared to Just Biohacking.

Part I. Awareness.

Chapter 1: Just Awareness.

X. The Intangibles Become Tangible.

XX. Everyone Has Infinite Flow Potential.

XXX. Release Emotional Holding Patterns.

XXXX. Detox With Methyl Folate, Especially for Those Who Do Not Have the Gene.

XXXXX. Mitochondria.

Chapter 2: Food.

X. Current Mass Food Production.

XX. Food Choices.

XXX. Dr. Zach Bush & His Ion Biome.

Bliss Intake.

X. Food Pairing Guide to Burn More Fat as Fuel.

Drink.

X. Mountain Spring or Spring Water.

XX. Optimal Hydration.

The Heart.

X. Ambidexterity.

XX. Michael Gelb.

XXX Whole Body Whole Brain Program Stems From Decades of in the Trench Experience With Our ATHLETICISM Programs.

Chapter 3: Nerve Health, Stress & Stressors.

X. Light Therapy and Stacking the Nervous System.

XX. The Schumann Resonance.

XXX. Things That Downregulate the Nerves.

XXXX. How to Rid Stressors, Including EMF.

XXXXX. Emotions and How They Play a Role With Chronic Stress & Overall Nerve Health.

Part II. Whole Body Coordination.

Chapter 4: Whole Body Exercises.

X. Coordination, Ambidexterity, Rhythms.

XX. Cross Crawl.

XXX. Jonathan Niednagel.

XXXX. PGA, ATP, AVP, and MLB.

XXXXX. Components to Whole Body Development.

Methods & Intangibles.

X. Non-Sport Specific.

XX. Flow & Coordination.

XXX. Peter Smith.

XXXX. The Figure 8.

Building a Solid Foundation.

X. Joint Stability and Integrity for Foundational Strength.

XX. Progression.

Breathing.

X. Pavel Kolar.

XX. Foundation Development.

XXX. Pedram Shojai, Brian MacKenzie, Richard LaPlante, Wim Hof & Troy Casey's System Strategies.

Chapter 5: Speed Techniques.

X. Learn How to Run.

XX. Move With Cross-Crawl Patterns.

XXX. Progression.

XXXX. Warm-Up.

XXXXX. Stride Length.

XXXXXX. Running Techniques.

Speed & Coordination Drills.

X. Figure 8's & Semicircles.

XX. Running, Skipping, Bounding & Shuffling Drills for Coordination.

XXX. Progression to Speed.

Part II. Whole Body Coordination.

Chapter 6: Power.

X. Knee Drives, Barriers & Power Running.

XX. Power Jumping.

XXX. Dot Drills.

Chapter 7: Olympic Lifting for Sports & Squats.

X. Coach Jerzy Gregorek.

XX. Foundation Lifting With Body Weight

XXX. Proper Body Weight Squatting Techniques.

Chapter 8: Stretching.

X. Active Isolated Stretching (AIS) for Sport, Life, Recovery, Injury Prevention & Ridding Stiffness.

Chapter 9: Balance Development.

X. Balance Progressions.

XX. BOSU, Dyna-Disc, Gym Ball, Extreme Balance Board.

XXX. The Figure 8 Board & Movement System.

Chapter 10: Kettlebells.

X. Steve Cotter & IKFF.

XX. Proper Swings & Benefits.

Part III. Whole Brain Coordination.

Chapter 11: Whole Brain Exercises.

X. Components to Whole Brain Coordination and Development.

XX. Beta, Alpha, Theta, and Delta Brain Waves.

XXX. Brain Entrainment With HeartMath & MindSpa.

XXXX. Ambidexterity Exercises & the Science Behind Eye-Hand Exercise.

Cup Stacking.

X. Stacking Cups to Develop Soft Quick Hands, Relaxed Concentration, Ambidexterity, Processing.

XX. Perform Under Timed Situations.

Juggling.

X. The Sequence to Learn Juggling 3 Balls.

XX. Increase Difficulty With Neuro Stacking…Doing More Than One Thing at a Time.

XXX. Learn How to Juggle 4 Balls.

Washers/Poker Chips.

X. Learn Ambidexterity Sequences of Tossing Up Quarters, Poker Chips & Washers.

Dexterity Strength.

X. Develop Finger and Hand Strength & Coordination.

Part III. Whole Brain Coordination.

Chapter 12: Eye Speed & Reaction Development.

X. Beads.

XX. Cross-Eye Method.

XXX. Light Therapy.

XXXX. Montak Chia's Qi Gong Exercises.

Chapter 13: Games & Ambidexterity Exercises.

X. Writing, Drawing & Coloring With the Opposite Hands.

XX. Kicking With the Opposite Foot.

XXX. Stay Balanced on Each Side.

XXXX. Dribble With Both Hands & Feet.

Conclusion: The Infinite Flow.

X. Live for Life.

XX. Find the Infinite Flow of the Universe Through a Proper Intake, ATHLETICISM, Ambidexterity Development & Figure 8 Movement Systems.

XXX. The 3 Pillars.

Gratitude.

Thank you to my family, friends, and colleagues.

Foreword.

Jason Cabell, 20-Year Retired Navy SEAL
Hollywood Writer / Director / Producer
Huge accolades for Justin Frandson and this book.

Justin is a consummate pro. He is an innovative pioneer and always one step ahead. After 20 years as a Navy SEAL, I have worked with the best when it comes to therapy, rehab, and training. Justin's nerve work and whole body, brain coordination were things I had never seen. His adaptive stretching and treatments have brought me closer to restoring function, faster than anticipated. His creative, out-of-the-box approach is refreshing and effective.

The injuries I sustained serving our country in combat led me through numerous surgeries and are ever-present. The treatment and exercises Justin provided for me have brought immense comfort.

When watching him do athletic development and coordination with my 14-year-old son, I saw the brilliance of his science at work. Justin's understanding of multi-disciplines shined, and I could tangibly see my son becoming more coordinated after just a few sessions.

There are few in the industry that have a background working with Navy SEALS to PGA pros. Justin and his ATHLETICISM program do it seamlessly. To my knowledge, Justin's

ATHLETICISM program offers one of the only whole body, brain, ambidexterity approaches in the business. His sensory nerve treatments for acute vision and spatial awareness double as concussion treatments. He uses light, sound, and your own coordination to optimize performance.

Justin has my highest recommendation. I am honored to be a client and call Justin my friend. I know you will enjoy his book, as it is everything and more that I have seen and experienced. Implement it into your daily life and get incredible results.

Prologue.

Most every sports enthusiast marvels at the greatest performers and how they consistently stay at the top of their game. Athletes strive for it. Whether you are part of a team or individually looking to dramatically improve your performance, this *ATHLETICISM* book will give you the stepping stones to elevate your game with that same consistency and flow of the greatest players, teams, and dynasties of all time. No matter your exercise, activity, sport, or level, your performance will significantly improve through our ATHLETICISM methods.

This is the *one* book to read to learn how to get into a universal rhythm, so you can become a Whole Body and Whole Brain performer. Simply put, I will teach you the trade secrets the pros use. I share in-the-trenches experiences and stories of athletes and teams, uncovering their growth and countless learning experiences. It will excite your interest to read the extensive research from top doctors and industry experts. I have seamlessly compiled decades of knowledge with actual protocols to follow. If you ever wondered how ambidexterity plays a role in performance, this book not only shows you, but will teach you how to become more ambidextrous to improve your own performance.

Unless they are racing the clock from point A to B, athletes don't move in straight lines when competing. My teaching has always coupled that philosophy, bringing us to train in semicircles and figure 8's. Are you looking for more energy, speed, and improved performance? Are you stuck at a certain level and want to improve? Are you searching for a new protocol to take your game to another dimension? Then this is the book you have been searching for with all the answers. It will unlock your Whole Body and Whole Brain to more connections and coordination. In turn, it will help develop you into a significantly improved version of yourself.

ATHLETICISM covers three distinct pillars:

1. Developing More Awareness.
2. Whole Body Exercises.
3. Whole Brain Exercises.

The first pillar, Awareness, covers the use of proper semantics, having an optimal food intake, and eliminating stressors. We enter the conscious and subconscious realms to clear away the old and create the new. When your energy on the inside and outside is flowing, your body and brain do, too. This is the same with optimal health and nutrition. They directly correlate to the sharpness of your body and mind, so you can enter the superconscious state. It is all about amping up the frequencies of your body to heal and thrive. I will show you how to achieve this unbridled awareness and energy.

The Whole Body Exercises section takes us back to the root of movement using cross-crawl patterns in various rhythms and figure 8 coordination. We use the beginning skipping, jumping, and shuffling movements for improving coordination. We show how to increase speed, spectrum, and intensity to develop top end speed for more advanced performers. The fun factor is that these movement systems rack your brain and make the most gifted athletes feel uncoordinated. Appropriately challenging the coordination of the Whole Body develops your brain's plasticity and ties directly in with our Whole Brain programs. With more connections from the brain to the body, performance exponentially improves.

This brings us to our Whole Brain Exercises section where we learn countless eye-hand exercises. We teach ambidexterity as the focal point for developing the brain. We have specific exercises to take you into optimal brain wave states. We have specific eye exercises to train the muscles of the eye. This is one of the most comprehensive brain development programs available.

All amateur athletes, professional athletes, weekend warriors, doctors, trainers, therapists, parents, active sports enthusiasts, strength coaches, and industry practitioners will see instant, tangible benefits within themselves, their kids, or their clients. Many of the benefits you'll find in this book include but are not limited to:

- Developing a deeper awareness to increase your health and performance
- Improving the quality of your food intake and your gut microbiome

- Ridding yourself of unwanted stressors
- Learning an entire foundation program
- Developing speed, coordination, power, and ambidexterity to run faster, jump higher, and change directions quicker
- Take-home protocols for stretching, strengthening, warm-up, and recovery to improve performance, prevent injuries, and rid stiffness from an injury state
- Learning about ATHLETICISM Neuro Stacking and how it quantifiably gets you about 20% stronger instantly
- All this and much more…

Combining multiple exercises together at the same time is called ATHLETICISM Neuro Stacking. It stresses your nervous system appropriately, so you make gains. We have success stories from countless athletes showing how our ATHLETICISM athletic development programs facilitated in elevating their performances. Even though you are genetically predisposed and brain typed a certain way, implementing our programs will remap you, elevating your performance beyond your genetic wiring. Our programs can create endorphin releases that feel amazing, and the results are undeniably quantifiable. This program develops pure ATHLETICISM at its finest. The definition of Athleticism is:

"The quality of being coordinated and physically strong while also having stamina and coordination. Physical prowess consisting variously of coordination, dexterity, vigor, stamina, etc. A show of athletic prowess."[1]

I have a strong desire to improve the awareness of the masses, apply my 23+ years of professional experience in the sports performance, fitness, and health and wellness industries. This gives you the ultimate road map of advantages for Whole Body Whole Brain development. All this, with body and brain nutritional information, can impact your life in the most positive manner. The human body and mind have abundant potential, even though we may feel a certain limitation from our genetic makeup. When we realize a higher level of awareness and consciously tap into exercises that connect us to the infinite flow, we can be, do, and create anything.

My message is simple and consistent: to achieve unbelievable results, develop your whole body and whole brain through awareness, coordination, figure 8's, nerve work, and ambidexterity. This will elevate your performance.

Although it's a simple message, together we will dive deep into how. We have an awareness that far surpasses the norm, and we will share it with you. Until now, there is not one book in the health and performance lane that lays out the road map of becoming ambidextrous to elevate your game. We

---

[1] YourDictionary.com

take the intangibles and make them tangible. We will teach you how to sync the right and left hemispheres of your brain. We get instant results, and your performance will show it.

....

Justin Frandson, APC, CPT, is an ATHLETICISM Performance Coach (APC) and founder of Athleticism.com and EMFRocks.com. Over the past 2 decades, he and his ATHLETICISM protocols have touched the lives of an endless list of clients, many of whom are playing or have played professional sports on the PGA Tour, NFL, MLB, NHL, AVP, WSL, and NBA. He has an impressive corporate clientele, YPO clients, SEALs, and is known for getting fast results. He currently has a successful sports performance, sound therapy membership, and concussion recovery practice in Newport Beach, California, where he treats and develops athletes and individuals of all ages and levels through nerve work, sound, light, and frequency, via ATHLETICISM Neuro Stacking.

In the Trenches.

Similar to our genetic makeup, we are all born with a predetermined brain type, says brain expert, Jonathan Niednagel. According to his research, we are all wired in 16 different ways. We can tell how we are individually wired by how we behave, move, answer questions, and handle stress. Some have more energy in crowds and are labeled extroverts. Some have more fine or gross motor skills. Others have more spatial awareness. Some are better suited for playing offense or defense, even filling specific positions because of their intuition or feeling, judging, or perceiving wiring. Much of this brain typing research came from Myers-Briggs and was modified by Niednagel who explores athletes' brain types and shows how to use that information to facilitate their awareness for success.

The questions that inspired me to write this book are: How do we elevate our innate brain and body type to excel at the highest level in our chosen endeavors? How do we develop our body and brain to capture our infinite potential? How do we overcome the stressors (emotional, biochemical, or physical) that are slowing us down?

The answers lie within this book in the 3 pillars for human performance:

1. Develop conscious and subconscious awareness

2. Whole Body exercises
3. Whole Brain exercises

Before we continue with a more detailed explanation of the pillars, it's important for you to have a reference point about the history and origin of the programs you will be reading about in this book. Our programs and these concepts have deep roots in athletic development in amateur and professional sports from pioneer and my mentor, Dean Brittenham. Dean has paved the way for us, working with many of the greatest athletes and teams during his era, including the University of Nebraska, Indiana Pacers, Baltimore Orioles, the Williams sisters, Jim Currier, Todd Martin, Steve Finley, Adrian Gonzalez, CC Sabathia, and many more.

My first experience with legendary coach Dean Brittenham was in the summer of 1998. His son Greg was the strength and conditioning coach for the NY Knicks NBA team. Back then, there was neither a summer league nor anything for the players to do during the summer. Greg wanted his team to make gains and scheduled them to take a trip to La Jolla, California, to our facility at Scripps Clinic.

One of the NY Knicks players on the team was Scott Brooks. Scott and I had a great rapport during the short time they trained with us. I lost touch with all the players for years once they left. One Saturday morning, about a decade later, I played against Scott Brooks in a recreation basketball game. We did not recognize each other until after the game. Reconnecting as long-lost friends, we ended up developing a friendship that has lasted over the years and have worked together again. I even had his son as a client.

In 2018, I went back to the NBA Summer League to see Scott Brooks, who had become head coach of the NBA's Washington Wizards. Prior to the game, we chatted for a bit, then I sat to watch his game, and one of the wildest things happened. When I sat down, there was one Wizards' credentialed guy near me. At the NBA Summer League, they have open seating and every NBA team staff wears credentials. Within a few minutes, the entire front office of the Washington Wizards was sitting around me.

We all said hello, and I shared that I knew their coach, Scott Brooks. They asked how, and I proceeded to tell the story of the team coming to train with us when Scott played for the Knicks. One of the Wizards' management pointed to the guy sitting directly behind me and said, "He was general manager of the Knicks at that time." His name was Ernie Grunfeld. I turned around and asked Ernie if he knew Greg and Dean Brittenham. He said, "Yes, I hired Greg. I wanted to hire Dean, but Dean was with the Indiana Pacers and said his son would be a perfect fit." We talked the entire game. Greg ended up being the strength coach for the NY Knicks for about 25 years. To learn that I had earned Ernie's admiration, a former star professional basketball player and now, a long-term, successful GM for my mentor Dean, his son, and this entire program meant the world to me. He said he wanted to hire Dean because Dean was doing the most creative and cutting-edge drills he had ever seen.

This ATHLETICISM program has continued to grow with the most incredible protocols, all documented in this book. The wisdom and awareness of this program is so captivating, rudimentary, and advanced, all at the same time. It can make significant improvements to your performance in every aspect of life! It is meant to inspire and educate all to make simple changes in their life, with the awareness ahead of the times. Some of these concepts you may be aware of, but combining them with the entire approach provided here will garner tremendous results for you, your loved ones, and anyone to whom you recommend this book.

Diving in further, let's look at the adage of practice, practice, practice. Hustle and work ethic were my recipe for success, and I completely embodied them. I am an ENTP (Extrovert, Intuitive, Thinking, Perceiving) brain type, or what is now called FCIR (Front, Conceptual, Inanimate, Right-brained). This type currently has the greatest number of professional athletes in sports. It's considered one of the proper brain types to be a pro due to the thinking skills involved. I was very coordinated, but I fell well short of competing at the professional level. I played about 4 hours of tennis most days of the week for years but didn't come close to playing professionally. Relentless practice is great and is a big part of the puzzle, but if you don't have the fine motor skills, coordination, proper foundational strength, alpha brain waves, rhythms, or connections from your brain to your body to perform at a higher level, you are less likely to get to where you want to go. You are less likely to perform under timed, pressure situations. You are less likely to quickly elevate your performance to new heights.

This is especially true when you are just doing the same repetitive motions again and again. So, only practicing longer won't get you to your highest potential, and it won't get your brain waves in the optimal flow state. Perfect practice does not exist if your coordination, brain wave entrainment, and nerve health don't allow you to get there. The flow state needs to be cultivated off the court with brain wave entrainment and coordination development. Our Whole Body Whole Brain program will provide you with endless exercises to seamlessly develop and open these pathways to performance at the highest level you can achieve. This will not only save your body from repetitive injuries, it will also harness your development in exponential ways.

The roots of developing more connections from the brain to the body entail becoming more ambidextrous with your lower and upper body. The essence of improving performance includes getting the brain to develop more energy in other parts that were not originally wired to fire. The Whole Body and Whole Brain sections of this book provide exercises that will get you there. You will initially feel like the most uncoordinated person when doing many of our exercises.

Challenging your coordination reveals a few of the keys to improving your performance with our Whole Body Whole Brain exercises. This development will add a new dimension to your game. You will no longer telegraph your next move, and your creativity will shine.

Having been in the trenches with endless athletes, teams, and corporations at every level, I have seen firsthand that being a Whole Body Whole Brain performer undeniably improves performance. The results are tangible with newfound coordination and ATHLETICISM, boosting rankings and increasing earnings.

One of the most creative thinkers who developed a monumental primal reflex nerve healing system is John Iams, PT, founder of Primal Reflex Release Technique (PRRT). John gave me an incredible testimonial in 2000 touting that, "Justin is a Coordination Mentor whose concepts are far ahead of his time." Thank you, John, for seeing early on the power of Whole Body Whole Brain development and teaching me the importance of nerves in performance exercises.

The increased awareness of optimizing your delta, theta, alpha, beta, and gamma brain wave state is another huge part of performance. We will show you how these ambidexterity and Whole Body Whole Brain programs get these levels into the desired state. This awareness also ties into what and how you feed your body with rest, exercise, hydration, and nutrition. It is so difficult to make massive headway when your body feels off, or you have brain fog, sinus pressure, muscle aches, tired eyes, pains, you're carrying extra weight, you might even have a leaky gut, or your adrenals may be shot.

An impressive number of experts have helped to shape our program. Their backgrounds range from track and field, stretching, strengthening, Olympic lifting, acupuncture, chiropractic, orthopedic doctors, physical therapists, massage therapists, nutritionists, homeopathic doctors, eye doctors, brain specialists, kinesiotherapists, inventors, kettlebell experts, masters of chi energy, mental coaches, and shamans. I am blessed to have interviews with most of them on GoBeyondSummit.com. Their diverse backgrounds opened my eyes to a new thought process in developing the Whole Body Whole Brain program to the fullest.

Once our three pillars of performance are addressed, you will have the program to tap into your full potential in ways you may have only dreamed of achieving. This book explains a comprehensive, proven system that crosses over into every sport and activity to take your performance beyond your expectations. This book is a lifestyle concept with direct exercises to support your efforts in preparing for competition. Once you are informed about how to apply these concepts, exercises, and nutrition, you will prepare smarter by doing minimal work, for maximum results and longevity.

Whole Body Whole Brain work is non-sport specific and non-activity specific. No matter your endeavor or ability level, your performance will elevate because coordination development is cerebral work. This is an entire book to drive your overall nerve, heart, soul, and brain health. So again, why Whole Body Whole Brain? In everything we do, we believe in challenging the status quo. We develop systems and treatments that show amazing, instant results. We just happen to work at the deepest level with the brain and nerves, facilitating in supporting athletes and individuals to become stronger, more flexible, and get them out of pain, allowing them to thrive.

I hope this sparked your attention. Are you ready to start thinking creatively? Are you ready for a lifestyle shift for boundless energy? Do you want to get fast? Are you ready to challenge your coordination, rhythm, and brain plasticity? Are you ready to find the infinite flow and elevate your performance to unlimited levels? Let's do this!

Background.

Most people's living experiences shape and define their lives. I was raised on mac and cheese and Kentucky Fried Chicken (KFC). I ate Barone's pizza (still amazing) and frozen, non-organic green peas for veggies. Yes, toast with extra butter and milk at every meal, especially before bed. I also drank about half a gallon of milk or more every day, mostly straight out of the jug. I assume it will sound like the diet of most average Americans who grew up in the 1970s and 1980s with bread, fried foods, pasta, milk, butter, and cheese as staple items.

Although I had the same food intake as much of the population, my father's hustle and hard work had paid off. My parents could afford to humbly provide me with private coaches. I had the advantage of a tennis court in my backyard. I felt I was unique in the sense that I had a more aware, emotional IQ than the average person. I was not fazed by fluff, watches, or cars. Instead, I surrounded myself with doers and positive role models. I always followed my intuition and searched for answers to performing at a higher level. There is not one reason I should not have played D1 college sports. So, why did someone like me not elevate my play to the next level as I felt I should? This book is fueled by a lifetime of hard learning, with several defining moments. It started as a food allergy.

Much of our society was focused on fitting in and promoting what was already popular in our culture. When I was growing up, practically everyone I knew ate cake, ice cream, and cupcakes at birthday parties. But I realized early on that, when I ate those things, I could taste how fake they were, and I didn't feel well after I ate them. My Mom never rewarded me with sweets, so I never acquired a sweet tooth.

But, what do you do when you get a stomachache and don't feel well after you eat? What if your energy is shot? You feel brain fog? You gain weight? You get sick or injured? You have sinus pressure? You have a constant low-grade sore throat? You have dark bags under eyes?

Most people eat unhealthy foods because they taste great, and many are staple foods of our culture. Plus, many of us are rewarded with these sweets as treats. Yet, somehow, there is minimal awareness of the health factor and detoxing needed. Maybe it is because our bodies are so resilient and overall, most don't consider the long term, cumulative effects? If it is sold in a market, it is food. I fell into that category of thinking during my youth, with the exception of sweets. I would flat out eat most of an entire large pizza then curl over on the couch for 30 minutes with a massive stomachache. I thought it was because I ate too much, not because I was allergic to the food (wheat and dairy). I was even eating healthier than most kids I knew.

Eating foods you don't assimilate has an instant negative effect on your performance. It can limit someone from being the best they can be. I have learned there is a more aware approach to health, and I can't wait to share my secrets.

I considered myself an athlete, gaining a varsity letter in both soccer and tennis as a freshman in high school. From what my parents said and fed me, I thought my intake was balanced and would bring me to greatness. My Dad taught me patience, mental toughness, hustle, and work ethic. I enjoyed tennis and spent hours on the court every day. My private coaches had me hit balls over and over again and ran me into the ground. I was tough as could be and had boundless energy. I had excellent tennis coaches, but I received no real performance cues with substance and no nutrition advice to raise me up into new levels. It was about just hitting balls, putting more time in on the court, and thinking maybe I would get good. It was ingrained in me to be this one-dimensional athlete.

As far as I knew then, I was eating lots of yummy food, providing fuel to my body, and working out, so I thought I was doing what I was supposed to do. Subconsciously, my body kept telling me, "What in the world are you doing eating food you can't digest, are allergic to, and why are you beating the crap out of me?" Thick white coating on the roof of my tongue, bad breath, rancidity, stomachaches, extra body fat, body odor, athlete's foot, and very little muscle or muscle tone. I was a mess, and most would never know it. I did not even realize it, because I did not know how to listen to my body, nor did I know an easier way at that time.

Looking back on my poor food intake and shortfalls of achieving athletic greatness, there are 3 pivotal learning experiences that shaped my pursuit of helping others. First, when I was 7, my father got a staph infection in his spine. To save his life, the doctors operated on his spine, removing the staph, paralyzing him, and giving him a lifetime of neurological challenges. Second, I developed several injuries (both wrists and my left knee), taking me out of soccer and tennis during my senior year. Third, the following year I got sick, with a weakened body, due to electromagnetic radiation (EMF) from sleeping in an apartment with a powerline generator outside my wall. I had kissed a girl who had mono 6 months prior, and she was still getting it out of her system. Since my immune system was weak from my intake and EMF exposure, the introduction to the frequency of mono was too much for my adaptive immune response to handle. I got mono that turned into Epstein-Barr virus (EBV). This series of events drove me to find answers, and I wanted to share what I learned so no one else would have to go through what I did. Each of these events resulted in my missing out on years of health, sports, fun, and love.

Studying Business (Entrepreneur emphasis) and Exercise Science at the University of Southern California (USC), I could not put my finger on what specific direction I wanted to move forward in after I graduated. I was constantly searching.

I even went to my cross-town rival, UCLA, and got my Emergency Medical Technician (EMT) certification my senior year. All three of my major learning experiences occurred before I graduated college, so I was already seeking answers and a specific direction. The doctor who fixed the slight tear in my medial collateral ligament (MCL) from my soccer injury, along with many other injuries, Wing Hsieh, taught me all about acupuncture and his cross-friction massage techniques. He was an MD from China who came to the US, doing a combo of acupuncture and cross-friction massage. He is now retired but had an amazing practice in Beverly Hills. I became highly proficient at his cross-friction massage techniques for getting rid of injuries.

Dr. Stephen Stiteler, in Santa Monica, was the guy who brought me back to life after I had mono. He taught me about applied kinesiology (also known as muscle testing), nutrition, acupuncture, and holistic/homeopathic medicine. I will never forget my first visit to his office when I was so sick. I thought I was the coolest and toughest kid who knew it all. As he sat across from me, he started muscle testing me using his fingers, verifying each time with vials of the actual viruses. He wrote down a list of things I was allergic to and should avoid. It was the wildest thing I had ever seen. At that moment, I was highly skeptical and had never seen anyone do energy work like that before. I came home and shared with everyone what I had experienced. They started calling him the voodoo doctor. The next day I felt remarkable! I made the changes he asked for, and the results were instantaneous. My sinuses started flushing like a river, and my body started flowing and filling with energy again. He brought me into the next best version of myself.

Even before I got mono, those constant stomachaches, bad breath, and baby fat were signs that I ignored to a certain extent. At one point, my stomach pain escalated so much that I got a stomach scan to make sure there was nothing wrong with me. It was a relief to know there was nothing to worry about with my stomach. The doctor said it was "just gas" and gave me zero ways to resolve it.

I now realize that the gas was a major sign of an intake that did not agree with me, but the medical doctor gave me no credible or tangible solution. Thanks, doc for the radiation in the stomach and gas diagnosis. I thought, "Now what do I do?" That literally drove me to keep researching and thinking creatively. I realized the excess gas meant I was not assimilating my food efficiently because of my allergies. Even relatively clean intakes will produce gas, but not debilitating gas, unless there is an allergy to certain foods. The MD didn't think to check that.

I recently went back to Montak Chia's seminar in Los Angeles. He recommends pressing into your stomach to burp the excess gas out before you sleep. This exercise helps you sleep and digest. I wish I would have known this in my youth.

There were many good things that came from having minor health challenges at an early age. Dr. Stiteler taught me I was allergic to wheat and a variety of foods, which transformed me and my life path. This knowledge brought me to becoming a pioneer in the gluten-free movement. This and the other challenges drove me on a quest for learning and not just accepting the normal Western medical philosophy or our common cultural intakes.

I grew up in Southern California and thought the only way to get good was to play about 3 to 4 hours of tennis per day. I got decent at tennis but ended my competition at an early age due to wrist injuries. When I injured my wrist, my Mom took me to a wrist specialist in Beverly Hills, the best money could buy. He gave me a diagnosis of a "weak wrist." The doctor thought I was weak because I had never lifted weights. If my wrist was not injured, I could have crushed his hand with my grip strength from tennis. I really wanted to because he was no help whatsoever. I had spent the entire summer scooping ice cream and had unbelievably strong forearms. When you carry a racquet around for about 4 hours a day, your forearms get very strong, almost like Popeye's. There are 8 carpal bones and 5 metacarpal bones in the wrist. In retrospect, one chiropractic adjustment of my wrist would have allowed me to initiate the healing process. Playing nonstop with my carpals out of alignment, I developed deep tendon, ligament, and cartilage injuries. It was unfortunate that chiropractors were not in my realm at that time. Now they are one of my first go-to healers.

In college, I was 6'2", about 180 pounds, with a broad 35" waist, all from being athletic and playing lots of sports. I constantly tested my strength on my older brother who was 6'3" and captain of the water polo team at Chapman University. I was not the guy with the biggest muscles, but my Qi (energy) was very strong, I had athletic hustle and intuitive instincts. I took Tae Kwon Do at age 12 to13, and I became really flexible and learned how to harness my power, developing tremendous confidence. Coming up short from achieving athletic D1 collegiate and professional status, I learned that it was not my fault from lack of effort. I was at a disadvantage from my lack of strength, whole brain development, being linearly trained, and improperly nourished with lots of food that did not agree with me. Since I could run all day and kick a soccer ball with both feet, I assumed I was doing the right stuff, but my brain and body were far from being nourished physiologically. My ambidexterity was far from the level necessary to overachieve for my brain type.

My quest for learning became even more solidified after college when I soon found my amazing mentor, Dean Brittenham. Dean was a giant-hearted, brilliant mind and one of the pioneers in human performance. He was a performance, speed, and strength coach out of Scripps Clinic, Shiley Pavilion in La Jolla, California. His teachings shifted my life in the direction I had been seeking all those years. I was young with endless energy and did not want to be a bean counter in the weight room, counting reps of clients on weight machines, with fixed axes and fixed ranges of motion. Nor did I want to be stuck in a small, square room all day under fluorescent lights. I did not want to needle clients. I did not want to just tape clients. I did not want to only see clients post operation. I did not want geriatrics only. I did not want to disrobe clients and be a masseuse. I wanted to make athletes better athletes.

Dean provided a platform for me to find the answers to heal through smiling, laughter, and improving the body, inside and out, through a Whole Body Whole Brain approach. Within a few years, Dean retired, and I took over the program at Scripps and founded ATHLETICISM and Athleticism.com. I continued to grow the program based on Dean's foundation, building speed, whole brain, coordination, and ambidexterity protocols. I constantly added even more to the coordination aspect, bringing in a holistic approach to health, awareness, and body movements. The program already was unbelievable and adding to it made it even more powerful.

It's important that we focus on eye-hand coordination, soft, quick hands, slowing the game down when going full speed…so it feels like you are flowing at the speed of time, staying in each moment in a superconscious state. It is all about processing information and performing with fluidity under timed, pressure situations. This ATHLETICISM program is about learning dexterity, ambidexterity, rhythms, cross-crawl movements, and breathing patterns, all necessary in developing brain and body plasticity. When you flow in the moment, with a universal rhythm, your performance becomes exceptional.

This program has transformed the lives of many of the world's greatest athletes, teams, publicly traded companies, their executives, and countless individuals.

The first time I read an article in *The San Diego Union-Tribune* newspaper about Dean making athletes better athletes, I fell in love with the concept. When I saw the program, I was blown away by his creativity and aware approach to working with the body and brain. When I did the program, my dormant body came alive and I had the most fun ever. The program was a track-based program from his days as a track and field coach at the University of Nebraska. It has roots with rhythms, non-linear movements, explosiveness, biomechanics, engaging exercises, taught with a smile and lots of amazingly bad (excellent) jokes. One joke I recall is, "How do you get fast? You eat fast food."

Dean and I had the most diverse group of athletes. We had NFL Chargers, MLB Padres, pro volleyball players, junior national figure skaters, and amateur athletes in multiple sports. Some of the amateurs were far more coordinated and flexible in our drills than the pros. When you have a junior national figure skater next to an NFL Charger, things get hilarious. This drove the pros to want to get even better. Our program was and is so special. As fun as it is, it garners undeniable, instant results.

Dave Asprey wrote in *Head Strong* that you can improve the mind 5X. I'm a fan of his biohacking to get these significant improvements. I believe we can do even more when implementing Whole Body Whole Brain development and get to at least 10X! Yes, 1000% on energy, performance, financially, pain, memory, and connecting the conscious to the subconscious. We have only begun to tap into the powers within and beyond.

In working with professional athletes, most of their sport coaches are just looking for an approximate 1% improvement for an edge over their competition. The margins are so tight at that level. When we open them up and do Whole Body Whole Brain work, we can tangibly measure their increases of salary, or even a corporation's earnings, far surpassing their coach's expectations.

My nerve rehabilitation, restoration, and stability programs or ATHLETICISM Neuro Stacking gets about 20% more strength instantly in each part of the body. I have quantified that through an ARX machine. Can you imagine the cumulative effect over the course of weeks, months, and of several years? Now you know how we get to the 1000%. Compounding our nerve work gets you there fast. Nerve health and neuro fatigue are two of the most missed areas of athletic development, and they are rarely a topic of conversation. Nerve health is solely the focus of my practice in Newport Beach, California, for performance, recovery, prevention, and concussion recovery. I will dive more into nerve restoration and Neuro Stacking later in the book.

Although we can achieve instant results, really going beyond requires a lifestyle shift. That takes time and diligence. As seasoned and result oriented as I am, practicing what I preach for the past several decades, I am only utilizing a fraction of my healing potential. But I continue to learn and grow, getting more powerful with my passion each day. For me, developing and consulting athletes is the best thing in the world. I have found how to harness wellness, coordination, and Whole Brain thinking, self-testing everything first. My protocols and outlook are detailed later in this book for you, too.

When I saw a Shaolin monk once, he showed me how powerful I could become. He had spent his entire life building energy to be lethally powerful. When he worked on me, it was like I was literally getting zapped from a strong electricity source. It was one of the most incredible experiences of my life. Now, I am sure most of us don't want to become a monk, nor need to be that electric, but we all can utilize our Qi energy powers to strengthen our own body, mind, and spirit.

I continue to hone my craft, getting rid of all the stressors and developing my healing and facilitating gifts to the full potential. Much of my focus in my practice now is stabilizing and lengthening clients and using pain reflex release techniques. I also use The LifeLine Technique and others to do emotional clearings. The limbic brain stores memories making us have a compulsion of emotions. Not until the conscious meets the subconscious will we release emotional holding patterns. Often, just clearing an emotion will get rid of an injury.

The best part of it all is how effortless it is to incorporate into our daily lives, no matter our age. My two favorite sports activities to do now are surfing and basketball. Surfing is for fun. Basketball is for competing and getting the lead out, a different, necessary fun. When I first started doing the ATHLETICISM program in my mid-20s, I soon started accelerating in basketball, having more court awareness, speed, explosiveness, fewer turnovers, and scoring more. Sustained energy, newfound athleticism, and hops I didn't have as a one-dimensional soccer and tennis player. Being able to dunk a basketball was proof of my transformation. The more I honed my intake and Whole Body Whole Brain development, the faster and more explosively I played.

My warm-up routine sets the tone for my performance each day. When I wake up my Whole Body Whole Brain nervous system before I play, my game is sharp. Just a simple warm-up of stretching, balancing on one leg while juggling and skipping, allows me to play at a higher level. Consistently doing my ATHLETICISM programs for workouts, combined with these proper warm-ups, is the key to improved performance. When I did not train my Whole Body Whole Brain, especially before I played, I might as well have gone for a jog or just sat on the bench instead of competing, because my performance was just bad and lacked rhythm, connection, or flow. I felt clunky, could not make a single shot, or even jump explosively. It is that tangible. When you do the program, you thrive.

I continue to use these same esoteric techniques and more with thousands of my clients, making the intangible, tangible. These are people of all ages, levels, and interests. They range from kids to Fortune 500 companies and executives. Many are already performing at high levels, but all are looking to reach new heights.

If you are more of an artist or musician and not as athletic, this program will still be highly effective for you. This program challenges the most academic in the group. Whole Body Whole Brain development is non-activity specific, meaning no matter what you do, these methods will bring you to breakthrough performances. If you are coordinated, get ready to quickly elevate your skills beyond your wildest dreams. You don't need to spend $1,000 each month or more at a fancy biohacking lab or gym. This book will empower you to implement our exercises into your life to achieve your potential simply by challenging your coordination and using the opposite side of your body more often. The road map is here with information, products, and services. You will soon start observing more details and putting the program into tangible action.

How long will it take? Most have instant feedback after 1 or 2 sessions. John Cook hadn't won a PGA tournament for 10 years. In less than 1 month, about 7 sessions of ATHLETICISM Whole Body Whole Brain development, including sessions with Tim Brown, DC, to help his shoulder, he won again. He thought his playing career was over until we remapped his shoulder and brain with our Whole Body Whole Brain protocols. For the next several years, I was by his side as he went on to have a successful career on the PGA Tour Champions and ranked in the top 5 each year. I also had a Carlsbad high school pitcher increase the velocity on his fastball 7 mph in 8 weeks. Last season, my client dropped .08 off her 100-meter sprint in 8 weeks through our nerve work, light therapy, and stretching. She was doing too much track work, so I had to do more recovery and stability work, which allowed her to run faster.

Now you know some of my skill sets used on a day-to-day basis. This book seamlessly incorporates my protocols of health, nutrition, and exercise awareness to optimize performance.

Are you ready to get a taste of stepping out of your comfort zone? Our movements combine rhythms of drumbeats and are done in figure 8's. To my knowledge, we are still one of the only ambidexterity programs in the country, linking and stacking coordination movements and eye-hand coordination together. We actually have dozens of eye-hand exercises, many we will share in the back portion of this book under the Whole Brain Exercises section. These exercises create an entire new chemical makeup in your body, so you release endorphins, norepinephrine, serotonin, and hormones that encourage performance.

It's time to jump into our 3 pillars.

Part I. Awareness.

Chapter 1: Just Awareness.

There is really one word that describes what we need in order to become more of a Whole Body Whole Brain thinker: awareness. Developing awareness of what to see and how to tap into your Whole Body Whole Brain is the secret recipe. This awareness is what we should all strive to achieve. The awareness of how to listen to your body, exercise in creative ways, raise your level of consciousness, get rid of stressors, boost your energy, and ground yourself at a deeper level.

I always wanted *Perfect Health* yet never felt I could achieve it, even after reading Deepak Chopra's book. I wanted to play collegiate tennis. Unfortunately, as I mentioned, I got hurt and sick prior and never had a chance to fulfill that dream. I was a product of the system and our culture. There were so many signals guiding me to the aware decisions, but it wasn't until my own lack of health forced me to make a change that it happened.

Just like every average all-American kid, I, got mercury fillings for cavities. I had every immunization shot they gave. I had aluminum in my deodorant and toothpaste. I drank out of aluminum cans. I grew up in the San Fernando Valley, which did not have the cleanest air quality. I was about 20 miles (too close) from the Simi Valley nuclear disaster. A pure valley boy, but at least I learned how to surf. After my soccer games, I would have trouble breathing from the smog. I drove countless miles on the 405 freeway in massive traffic with the windows down and music blasting. I graduated from USC in downtown Los Angeles, considered some of the worst air quality around.

After college, I traveled to Indonesia on a surf trip. Prior to the trip, I got tetanus, typhoid, and Hepatitis A shots. I was sick for 2 weeks before I left from the toxicity in the shots adding to my already toxic body. I just wanted to feel great, but every time I went to the medical doctor, I got worse?!

Through this education process, I learned that varying percentages of the population do not methylate properly due to mutation of the gene or genes, or they lack the proper coding of 5-methyltetrahydrofolate (5-MTHF). Without the proper coding, your detox mechanisms run at half speed, at best, so your energy and other systems will be compromised. Very few people even talk about this! In *Dirty Genes* by Ben Lynch, ND, and *Peak* by Marc Bubbs, ND, both speak about the challenges of not being able to methylate[2] or detox properly. A genetic mutation of this enzyme may result in extra toxicity from heavy metals, radiation, or other sources. In this situation, some immunization shots may overload your system and potentially cause tremendous health challenges.

---

[2] Bubbs M. *Peak: The New Science of Athletic Performance That is Revolutionizing Sports.* Chelsea Green Publishing; 2019.

For a simple and cost-effective fix, get some methyl folate at any health food store and increase your leafy greens. You must do it for the rest of your life. Many B vitamins have methyl in them as well, but most people don't know about this, and for the longest time, I was one of them. I can typically see in someone's eyes if they methylate properly or not. Darker circles under the eye are one indication they aren't, along with a lesser tolerance for alcohol.

Being aware of how to heal includes working with all aspects of the body. Let me give a simple example of making a more aware choice when it comes to quickly healing an injury. When someone sprains his or her ankle, the old method of healing was to rest, ice, compress, elevate, and let time heal it. Some of the most reputable doctors currently give casts and crutches and subscribe to this passive method of healing a sprained ankle. We feel this method is for a bygone day and age because now there is so much that can expedite healing.

Active healing, rather than just letting time mend the injury, is a more effective and aware approach to speeding up the healing process. Massage, stretching, acupuncture, arnica, Wobenzym or resveratrol (both are natural anti-inflammatories), chiropractic treatment, cold laser, heat, ice, light, sound, frequency healing, and more are numerous ways to start the active healing process! Yes, light is one of my favorites. Why would we be passive when the body responds so well to nutrition, touch, light, and love? Light therapy is replacing much of the ice, heat, and electrical stimulation.

This active approach should be taken even when doctors have to cast a severe fracture.

One of my clients was a two-sport, D1 athlete at the University of Southern California. He was such a high performer, and he wanted to get even better. He went to his mom and said he wanted to focus even more. His mother had no clue what to do, so she directed him to see their medical doctor. The doctor, of course without hesitation, prescribed him Adderall (Ritalin is also a popular go-to for doctors). These are popular drugs for doctors to prescribe for focus and attention challenges. Thank goodness my client called me on the way to pick up his prescription. I had worked with him for years and worked with his entire high school team. He had developed a strong respect for me.

He let me know what had transpired about wanting better focus. I said, "Before you consider taking a drug to get you to focus better, let's read the side effects, which are 'actual effects.' " The pharmaceutical companies just take one of the effects and highlight it. They call the others 'side effects,' but they are all effects. I continued to say, "You are at a pivotal point where you are about to take over the starting position and take your team to the D1, NCAA Finals." The effects of the prescription drug he was thinking of taking were listed as:

- nervousness
- restlessness
- excitability
- irritability

- dizziness
- headache
- fear
- anxiety
- agitation
- tremor
- weakness
- blurred vision
- sleep problems (insomnia)
- dry mouth or unpleasant taste in the mouth
- diarrhea
- constipation
- stomach pain
- nausea
- vomiting
- fever
- hair loss
- loss of appetite
- weight loss
- loss of interest in sex
- impotence
- difficulty having an orgasm
- increase blood pressure
- increased heart rate
- heart palpitations[3]

How do these effects improve performance? The doctor did not bother to share any of them with my client or his mom. Even if some of these effects happened only in a smaller percent of the population, this entire list was extremely frightening. It was like reading him the script of a pharmaceutical commercial where they list all the negative effects. Negative is probably the nicest word to describe

---

[3] rxlist.com

them. These effects were devastating to read and hear. Many of the commercials even list death as an effect.

I was so proud of him. Even though he had an older sibling on it, he never took the prescription drug. His first direction was to clean up his intake. Next, we added Qi Gong, meditation, and brain wave entrainment, which earned him a starting position, beating out a highly touted phenom. As he took his team to the NCAA finals, I sat in the stands and cheered him on. Awareness and education are key. Just explaining to him how the body works was enough. He chose to make the changes and did them with a proper mindset, intake, and Whole Body Whole Brain development.

To bring your awareness to an even deeper level, the chemical reactions or frequencies of something you love versus something you ignore are completely different. Dr. Emoto[4] clearly shows this in his work. There is so much more movement of the cells and blood when touch, love, and the intent of healing is implemented. Active healing can expedite the recovery of an ankle sprain in half the time, from the doctor's prediction of 6 weeks, to actually 3 weeks or less, depending on the age of the athlete and severity of the sprain. This is the power of being aware. It's so simple and yet so powerful. This active method holds true for healing all types of injuries.

---

[4] Masaru E. *The Hidden Messages in Water*. Beyond Words Publishing, Inc.; 2004.

This book shares with you the gift in cultivating your health and Whole Brain development. It can be easily replicated for everyone. Awareness information may not be received all at once. For some, it may be more of a timed-release capsule as Santron Freeman calls it. When you are ready to be aware, the information is here for the taking.

Being in the trenches with athletes, teams, and corporations, it is in my DNA for me to pass on what I have learned from my studies, hands-on experience in anatomy, physiology, kinesiology, the brain, nutrition, the nervous system, and human development.

My wife, a creative genius herself, is the founder of the Twistband, a globally branded hair accessory company that she built and sold within 5 years. She made the new scrunchie famous, a Twistband hair tie that did not damage or leave a dent in your hair and doubled as a wristband. In 2018, she made waves and continues to in the clean beauty movement with her next company, CampoBeauty.com, a luxury essential oils/modern aromatherapy company. As co-founder, she has curated wild crafted and organic blends that are intoxicating. Influencers say they are addicted to her scent stories. Her price point is unbeatable. Campo essential oils are part of our go-to products for performance. Her Campo Beauty's Focus essential oil pulse point roll-on has natural focus benefits from the sandalwood tree, and it smells so good that I use it daily as cologne.

With all my wife's talent, success, and branding skill, she still marvels at the creativity she sees when I interact with our daughter. At an early age we saw that our daughter was right hand dominant. She would always reach, play, and throw with one hand exclusively. When we would play, I would show her it was ok to use the other hand, no matter the activity. I always rewarded her with huge praise, hugs, smiles, high fives, and pats on the back or a healthy smoothie, juice, or yogurt. These simple early teachings helped her become ambidextrous in many ways.

As a parent, if I did not teach her to use both hands and feet, she would still be left brain, right side dominant in her motor skills, even with us playing classical music when she was in the womb. I'll humbly admit my wife and I are very active and coordinated, athletic individuals, so it's not hard to assume that our daughter would follow suit. But, as our brain type shows, she would have had limitations, ones that I saw early on, if I did not open up those pathways. This process will work with any individual at any level. I'll explain more about brain typing below.

As we compare notes with other parents about our abilities during the same time periods, unanimously we see our daughter is definitely a 10X version of us at the same age. Ambidexterity can be taught to anyone at any age, as it is a learned skill. There are so many studies showing how brain plasticity is accelerated with youth and continues with age.

The early years of our life are when development occurs for our health, mapping, and establishing connections from the brain to the body. Although, these early years are so pivotal, it is never too late to grow. At any age, our brain needs more exposure than time to synthesize the information. It may take months to learn various skills, like juggling proficiently, but you will learn. Some people will pick things up much more quickly depending on their wiring and toxicity.

There are several different brain types: some athletes have better cognitive (thinking) skills, motor (coordination) skills, and spatial (vision) awareness. Understanding your brain and how to train yourself to develop better thinking, movement, and eye-hand coordination is essential to performance. You can develop an athlete to improve his or her processing and decision-making skills when under pressure situations through our ATHLETICISM programs of Whole Body Whole Brain development. When someone is wired for one area of his or her brain to fire more, developing the whole brain will balance it and strengthen the other parts. This balance will, in effect, open up more options for the athlete, transferring into superior performances. This rewiring of the circuitry provides better options under pressure, instead of defaulting to the way the original wiring was ingrained. Individuals, especially athletes, will no longer telegraph (show their move too early) before the key moment happens, and they are far less likely to choke under pressure.

Once the athlete has an awareness of what tightens under pressure, they can realize what they are doing and take counter measures. It is similar to going to the dentist and he tells you to stop grinding your teeth. You had no idea you were grinding your teeth. Then, as you pay attention, you will catch yourself and slowly break the habit.

I trained a PGA golfer who carried all his tension in his hands when he felt stress. We brain typed him and gave him the tip to relax his hand before a big shot. He could not believe I knew that was his challenge. He knew he gripped the club too tight, but he was never taught how to make a change. No one ever told him his tight grip was a characteristic of stress from how he was wired. Once he developed this awareness and made the change, his low scores started coming in and he had the best year of his career.

There are amazing products to support Whole Brain consciousness and heart coherence, like HeartMath. There are others, like MindSpa, that passively take you into a parasympathetic mode to either rest, recover, or focus through brain entrainment, with audio and visual stimulation. Then, there are the week-long programs, like 40 Years of Zen, that use similar stimulation and ridding subconscious holding patterns, leaving you in the highest state of alpha and theta. All will enable you to create more than ever and perform at a higher level.

Did you know your body consists mostly of water, light, and energy? These 3 things are unbelievable in their own right. Just over 60% of the human adult body is comprised of water. The brain and heart are composed of 73% water, and the lungs are about 83% water.[5]

Many say, including Darren Weissman, DC, in his first LifeLine seminar, that the human body is like a holograph of light, just like a rainbow. George Gonzalez, DC, wrote a book called *Holographic Healing,* and by using light, developed a nerve healing system for doctors called Quantum Neurology® Rehabilitation. Our cells communicate through light, similar to plants and the photosynthesis process of deriving energy. We call this biostimulation[6], biophotosynthesis, and photobiomodulation. Have you ever seen someone glowing with magnetic energy, looking so healthy? That glow is the cells in their body communicating through light. You can tangibly see it. They often have great coloring, and it's definitely not from a tanning booth. In contrast, when you see some elderly people, they look pale, feeble, and weak. Their cells show they are aging and the light is dimming. Cells communicate through light, and light is directly correlated with your health. It's also wild how our chakras match the same color sequence as a rainbow. The colors and sequence of red, orange, yellow, green, blue, purple, and indigo are an

---

[5] What Is the Average (and Ideal) Percentage of Water in Your Body? Undated. Accessed April 11, 2021. https://www.healthline.com/health/body-water-percentage#body-water-storage

[6] Hashme JT et al. Role of low-level laser therapy in neurorehabilitation. *PM R*. 2010; 2(12 Suppl 2):S292-305. doi:10.1016/j.pmrj.2010.10.013

incredible parallel. Now you know why some of the greatest minds in medicine look to light, more so than ice or heat, to heal.

"Nobody is quite sure how cells produce biophotons but the latest thinking is that various molecular processes can emit photons, and these are transported to the cell surface by energy carrying excitons. A similar process carries the energy from photons across giant protein matrices during photosynthesis." A growing number of scientists are convinced that cells are bathed in the pale fireworks of a biophoton display. Sergey Mayburov at the Lebedev Institute of Physics in Moscow believes, "Biophoton streams consist of short quasiperiodic bursts, which he says are remarkably similar to those used to send binary data over a noisy channel."[7]

Now, it is also easier to explain why my light therapy nerve treatments and having awareness are so effective. I see the light. Do you?

．．．．．．．．．．．．．．．．．．．．．．．．．．．．．．．．

Listening to your breath is a great start to practice "being" in the moment. Exercises, like juggling, force you to stay in the moment and not think about anything else. This focus takes you into a parasympathetic mode, which is where great

---

[7] Biophoton Communication: Can Cells Talk Using Light? MIT Technology Review Website. Published May 22, 2012. Accessed April 11, 2021. https://www.technologyreview.com/2012/05/22/185994/biophoton-communication-can-cells-talk-using-light

performers want to be. The exercises in this book will teach you simple ways to stay present and cultivate more pathways in developing yourself to be a healthy body, Whole Brain thinker, feeler, doer, and creator.

Clients often ask my opinion about what level of play they can achieve. It is their choice or free will as to how high they want to go, not mine. There is an infinite flow potential that is virtually untapped in every individual, team, and corporation. So many athletes limit themselves and have coaches, parents, or others who limit their potential. There are often subconscious limitations ingrained in them at early ages. The Cohn Health Institute in Costa Mesa, California, can clear those limitations with Neuro Emotional Technique (NET). The LifeLine Technique, and other applied kinesiology systems, are other clearing systems that I have used for years. These holding patterns affect upper limits as Gay Hendricks shares in his book *The Big Leap*. They also show up in slowing down the healing process in an injury. Injuries disappear after doing The LifeLine Technique with my clients. Even the John Iams' Primal Reflex Release Technique (PRRT) has primal emotional releases that work really well for injuries and pain.

Studying The LifeLine Technique since 2002, founder Darren Weissman, DC, feels, and I agree, that the universal healing frequency is *"Infinite Love & Gratitude."* He uses this as his technology in harmonizing the body. The beauty is that anyone can give themselves, any part of their body, or anyone else Infinite Love & Gratitude, and it feels amazing.

The key is to use the sign language and say it at the same time.

> **Say it 3 times out loud!**
>
> Infinite Love & Gratitude
> Infinite Love & Gratitude
> Infinite Love & Gratitude

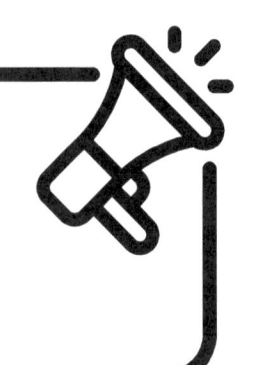

Place the hand sign for "I love you" on your heart when you say it. For clients and for myself, I use The LifeLine Technique to connect each day and night to my mind, body, spirit, and chakras. I also use it to ground myself more deeply to Mother Nature and connect myself to the Source. Each time you connect yourself to the mind, body, spirit, earth, and God, your energy is charged and your consciousness is elevated.

There are so many limiting beliefs where people just get stuck. Dr. Darren calls us "emotional junkies." The triune brain includes the limbic and reptilian brains that are more subconscious. These are the areas we will address now. We can be abundantly more productive to thrive to our full potential with this knowledge and practical application of having the subconscious meet the conscious.

John Iams' PRRT also has primal emotional release techniques. Tapping is another easy way for people to release these holding patterns. When I do any cranial nerve work or emotional work, I always check for cues that the patient is dumping and has sweaty palms. It is a sign of a sympathetic dump or nervous system overload. It is crazy to have someone with dry palms and have them do a primal emotional release. Their palms will get clammy wet instantly. They will have a euphoric floating or light feeling with the release. It feels like they just released the 1000 pounds they were carrying on their chest. It is incredible.

"Have some fun and don't forget to giggle," is what my friend, Energy Worker colleague and one of the greatest facilitators ever, Kent Ewing, advises. That is probably the best advice that can be given. In The LifeLine system, there is a clearing where people live for life or death. So, I always like to cue everyone to start living for life and enjoy the gift of presence with infinite love, light, blessings, abundance, prosperity, and gratitude!

Awareness includes a strong connection to God in your mind, body, and spirit. Once your mind, body, and spirit are connected to the Source, you will perform at a heightened state. This connection is one way to keep yourself in the moment, allowing you to see, feel, and do things others don't. Strong connections to God will allow you to manifest easier. This raises alpha levels from the fact that you are leading with your heart, not your head. The optimal alpha level will lead to more flow, especially in sports. It brings you to staying in the moment. This will not only help in your Whole Body Whole Brain development, but it will also allow you to connect to the flow state, moving toward optimal performance. Friend and Qi Gong expert, Jason Hanck, cued me in on this. He simply stated that the Source, God, loves you more than anything. When looking for more love and support, you know to whom to turn.

You want to stay in the parasympathetic nervous system of digesting and absorbing nutrients. Dr. Stephen Stiteler has a method called The Restorative Pose. Lay on your back with your feet up on a chair. Just close your eyes and breathe for about 15 minutes. It will feel as though you took a 45- to 60-minute nap. It will also help with low back pain as your leg length will balance out once your body is out of fight or flight mode.

Semantics and what you set as your intention have a lot to do with determining your outcome. Negative thoughts and words can limit achieving ultimate greatness and lower your frequency. Even the joking, self-deprecating words have an adverse effect. Each word carries a positive or negative frequency, affecting the body. I have garnered wisdom from many of the best mental coaches, including Mark Harradine, TheConsciousAthletes.com. They all agree that your positive thoughts, visualizations, daily writings, prayers, and repetition of each all set the intention for the universe to provide abundance. Reverse engineering where you want to be and bringing it to the now will facilitate in stronger manifestation and superior performance. Supporting this, Dr. Joe Dispenza wrote *Becoming Supernatural.* He also writes about blessing your chakras.

Since our body and mind don't know the difference between memory, reality, and imagination, they listen to everything we say. You won't hear me use the words try, can't, kind of, hard, or hate. Your body wants to hear words that are definitive, positive, strong, and full of action: I do, can, will. Instead of saying, "*Try* throwing it with your other hand," I would say, "Throw with your right hand. Now, throw with your left hand." The word "try" elicits a failure response before the action is even taken. One of my daughter's friends lost in a sport and she walked away singing, "I am a loser. I hate this and that." It was so wild to see and hear. My daughter heard her say it all, and at that moment she realized how powerful words are. The word "hate" has no room in our vocabulary. Also, if you are sick, don't take possession of the virus. It is not "my virus," it is "the virus." The proper use of semantics is huge. When you say something is hard, it really becomes hard.

Many of our society's greatest performers have been studied extensively. They are all asked about routines, journaling, goal setting, prayer, brain plasticity, imagery, and anything else they do that gives them an edge. There is unlimited data on the power of creating through consistency and repetition of the above. Once you have done that over and over, it, more often than not, becomes a reality.

When you are having fun, all systems are on go and the body becomes limitless. Brain expert and author Michael Gelb says, "The body has infinite possibilities with more pathways than atoms in the universe." The universe has an abundant flow that the individual needs to connect with when developing and performing. Gelb also states, "…the brain is so underutilized, that it can learn 7 facts per second for an entire lifespan and still have more room to learn."

One of the most effective ways to maintain health, energy, and one's composure during competition is to be thankful for each learning experience. Eaglewoman, one of my favorite shamans, is married to Sensei Benny 'The Jet' Urquidez. He is a famous former kickboxer who mastered having gratitude for each learning experience or shot to the face. He never lost a title fight in 62 fights. Watching replays of his fights on YouTube, you will see him in the middle of a fight, get hit in the face, smile, and essentially give the other fighter props, complimenting him for getting a great shot in. What a lesson in responding with appreciation and becoming an observer. When a bad call is made, even if the call was made only seconds ago, it is still in the past. We always teach to be grateful for that call and learning experience. The focus stays in the moment and on moving forward, not giving your power away to an opponent, referee, coach, or parent.

One of the largest cultural shifts we will see in the next decade is in people openly finding their Zen through meditation, Qi Gong, and breath work. These are my favorite ways to ground myself, stay in the moment, and move stuck energy. Lee Holden and Pedram Shojai, both Qi Gong masters, have incredible videos on how to build up your energy reserves and teach you how to breathe. I was in Pedram's first movie *Vitality,* and he also gave Athleticism.com a shout out in his first book, *Rise and Shine*. He recently produced his third documentary movie, *Prosperity*. Pedram is a gifted acupuncturist and is now on a massive movement for vitality and global sustainability. He teaches 100-day gongs to create a repetitive imprint in your body to make a massive change. You simply do the same routine every day for 100 days. You choose your routine each day and do it. One of my gongs was to do his Silk Weaver's routine. I have had multiple clients who held a plank position for several minutes every day. You pick your gong and create a new imprint in your body.

David Karaba, DOM, shared with me the idea of Cortisol Awakening Response (CAR). This means getting your cardio up first thing in the morning within 20 minutes of being awake. This entails spiking your heart rate to at least 70% of its capability for about 2 to 5 minutes. I love the sound of this. Did anyone else first think of morning intimacy, too? It makes a lot of sense. Just start your day by kicking it into deep breathing and the rest of the day is optimized. The CAR should be talked about more for weight loss and cardio health, as this ties in with our nitric oxide and anaerobic methods. I recommend setting your intentions prior to spiking your heart rate.

I pride myself on my creative approaches and thinking. I have always appreciated and respected people who do that as well. My Mom introduced positive visualization to my Dad when he was in critical condition after surgery removing a staph infection in his spine. As she would leave his hospital room, the nurses would always ask her, "What did you say to him? His vital signs normalize to such calm levels when you are with him, and they stay that way." Being positive and spreading joy, hope, love, and light is not so difficult. She also introduced him to acupuncture during his mending process. How many 7-year-olds in 1978 in the US saw acupuncture? I saw rooms of people lying down with needles all over their body. Deep inside me, I knew there was substantial merit. I could feel it.

Becoming a Whole Brain thinker will simply give you more opportunity to thrive in whatever you choose to do or be. You will be more creative, aware, alert, balanced, coordinated, and be able to process more information in a relaxed manner. I'm not one of those aggro parents who does things at all costs or expects their child to be the next legend in their favorite sport. I do, however, feel it is the parents' honor, privilege, and role to safely encourage, love, cultivate, and support their child's development. You will see the methods taught are seamless and full of fun common sense.

Have you heard of Infant Swimming Resource's (ISR) Self-Rescue program? The founder experienced a baby dying in just a few inches of water. He made it his life's mission to educate people that rolling onto our backs when we are submerged in water is a learned skill that can be taught at a young age. Google it. It is incredible to watch these infants with their instructors. They learn to fall into the water at every angle, float to the surface, and flip onto their backs to breathe. ISR teaches infants to become experts at back floating, even with their clothes and diapers on. Those extra minutes are the key to saving lives. These teachings continue to save thousands of children from drowning deaths annually. Whole Body Whole Brain development is also a learned skill set.

Keep in mind that, when your ATP production is on *"Go,"* you can be unstoppable. Your mitochondria will thrive when you properly feed your body and reserve systems. Your mitochondria are the powerhouses of your cells. The health and energy of your entire body and cardiovascular system depends on the cycle of ATP.

Remember hearing about the NFL players doing ballet? They were looking for more focus, balance, agility, coordination, flexibility, and fluidity. The thought process was headed in the right direction, but most athletes don't want to wear ballet clothes or tights and dance ballet. The other challenge is that dancers lead with their toes and athletes drive with their knees. So, although it helped in a lot of areas, they really needed a program designed for athletes. Now you have found it.

My wife inspired me to write this book and to share these creative approaches of our journey. We were blessed with the most incredible, healthy daughter. I make time to be an integral part of her coordination development. Outside of the thousands I have trained, my transformation and my daughter's transformations have been incredible. The best part is we are both starting at different levels and so can you.

The Heart.

The heart of this Whole Body Whole Brain program stems from ATHLETICISM (Athleticism.com), a human performance program for amateur and professional athletes, teams, and high-level corporate executive teams. This Whole Brain development is so scalable and versatile, it facilitates growth in virtually every scenario. Everyone, especially parents, can help facilitate the development of athletes and our youth with these exercises and concepts.

Look up the world's greatest athletes, and you will find they are all ambidextrous. Roger Federer, Tiger Woods, Lebron James, and the major super stars are whole brain thinkers. Even the geniuses of the world, including Leonardo da Vinci, were ambidextrous. We have found that ambidexterity development is the key to unlocking more pathways from the brain to the body. An excellent book that shares this philosophy is *How to Think Like Leonardo da Vinci* by Michael Gelb. Dean Brittenham found Gelb's work and contacted him. Dean always found the best ideas, and he started teaching athletes to juggle after reading Gelb's work. In his book, Gelb reveals the components of being a genius that we also follow. This list of a true genius includes:

1. Communication
2. Music
3. Art
4. Math and science
5. Kinesthetic awareness
6. Interpersonal
7. Intrapersonal
8. Vision[8]

Gelb impressed upon having interpersonal, intrapersonal skills, a keen, detailed artistic eye, kinesthetic awareness, science, math, verbal skills, and more. He says, "Leonardo trained himself to look at things other people passed over." Sounds like awareness to me. Leonardo felt a lot of his genius came from his ambidexterity work. He could paint with both hands. He juggled in his spare time. Juggling 3 balls by tossing them up to the other hand creates a figure 8 pattern. The figure 8 is the infinity sign. We want to connect to this rhythm and infinite flow. As performers, we want to put ourselves in a flow state, better known as "the zone." The more ambidextrous you can get your body and brain to

---

[8]Gelb MJ. *How to Think Like Leonardo da Vinci*. Dell Trade Paperback; 2004.

become, the easier it will be to connect with this flow state and stay in it. Thus, you will find a rhythm that is unstoppable.

Leonardo had an insatiably curious approach to learning. He was committed to testing knowledge through experience, persistence, and the willingness to learn from mistakes. He had a heightened awareness of all his senses and appreciated connecting with all things. What an incredible approach to life and cultivation of the Whole Body Whole Brain. When you feel good, you notice more things. You can be more creative and have energy to do more coordination exercises. You simply become better at what you do.

According to brain expert, Jonathan Niednagel and his son Jeremy, braintypes.com, there are 8 introvert and 8 extrovert brain types.[9] Each type predetermines how a human is wired from the brain to the body. Whether people are fine motor, gross motor, have more spatial awareness, or are language skilled, each has different strengths. This means there are numerous human tendencies regarding how people are wired and how they respond to certain circumstances, showing the most metabolic activity. Front vs. Back (extrovert / introvert), Empirical vs. Conceptual (sensing / intuitive), Inanimate vs. Animate (thinking / feeling), Left vs. Right Brain (judging / perceiving).

The key to this book is to understand that, no matter what the brain type is, it is important to develop areas of the brain

---

[9] Niednagel JP. *Your Key to Sports Success*. Laguna Press/Bti; 1997.

that people are less inclined to use on their own. This, in turn, makes the whole person stronger and more powerful. This is providing an aware approach of taking yourself out of your genetic wiring and challenging your coordination, thus allowing you to develop more pathways from your brain to your body. Brain experts, like Niednagel, acknowledge that being a well-rounded, Whole Brain thinker is what we want to strive for.

Now, you have a program to support this development.

I have found that many of the best athletes became significantly better when they became a Whole Brain thinker and performer. Under my care, Jordy Smith, a professional surfer, early in his career jumped to #2 in the world behind one of the greatest of all time, Kelly Slater.

Every ATHLETICISM exercise is designed to work both sides of your body, both hemispheres of your brain, both eyes, and connect them all together. It can be very challenging to learn. It often takes the best athletes in the world and makes them look so uncoordinated. It is that simple element of taking yourself out of your coordination comfort zone and stressing yourself appropriately that makes all the difference. Juggling is one of the exercises we do often. The rhythm, flow, and figure 8 is the foundation for ambidexterity. As you progress, we add new ways to juggle, or we add more balls and keep adapting.

ATHLETICISM

Chapter 2: Food.

The focal point of the program is to cultivate yourself to become a healthy Whole brain performer. Eating a proper intake will allow your brain and body to thrive. To simplify, we are teaching health in how to feed your body and brain.

The food we eat is a giant part that directly relates to energy production. Addressing what is transpiring in our mass food production will shed awareness on the massive amounts of modified and pesticide-laden food sold, which affects our health and energy. We have GMO foods, pesticides, artificial foods, preservatives, additives, dyes, steroids, hormones, artificial colors, depleted topsoil, demineralized water, over-salted foods, and we consume them at nearly every meal or snack. This is also fed to the food we eat. How are we supposed to be well and perform at a high level?

When I got sick at age 19, I initially saw several medical doctors. They put me on 4 courses of antibiotics back-to-back. Each prescription got stronger, only making me worse and weakening my bio-terrain. These doctors were supposed to be the best, but they were crushing me. Fortunately, my Mom had a progressive friend who referred us to Dr. Stephen Stiteler, a holistic doctor. He tested me for a variety of food allergies. The biggest allergy was to gluten in wheat. Imagine telling a stubborn teenager over 30 years ago to dramatically change his intake away from the norm. Since I needed to get my health and energy back on track, I reluctantly obliged and have not looked back. The choice I made to remove foods I didn't tolerate, including wheat and many staple foods, improved my health and energy. It brought a lot of skeptics to the surface, too. Wheat allergies were common in the US, yet very few people knew about them or knew anyone who had them.

I quickly learned that processed carbs were to be limited, eaten more as a treat or not at all, instead of several times a day as I had been. My father grew up on a farm in the Midwest with wheat as a primary source of food. So, even after I let everyone know I had a wheat allergy, I was still offered bread at every meal for over a decade. I am sure Novak Djokovic and I could have a few good laughs from going gluten free (GF). Everyone thought it was hilarious that I was allergic to a food that is everywhere and in almost everything. It got to the point that, to avoid embarrassment, I would just order a sandwich and peel the bread, eating it like a banana. I was already slender, so people would look at me like I was nuts. Lettuce wraps were not cool at that time. "Protein Style" did not exist on the menu. Several of my close friends also offered me bread at every dinner we had together. Now, we get a good laugh that they are GF, and so are their kids and pets.

It was a tough choice back then, but when I instantly realized I felt better without it, there was no question that I would make the shift. After college, I became even stricter about avoiding gluten and did not eat it at all. I continue to justify not eating wheat since I am more educated on the ingredients. Most people have no idea what manufacturers put in bread. Domino's and Subway, for example, were putting the worst ingredients in their bread. So, what is in the bread at markets or restaurants? You tell me if you're familiar with more than one ingredient on the label. In 2014[10], Subway and others were under tremendous pressure because they had the chemical *azodicarbonamide* in their bread. That chemical is used in making yoga mats. Also, now the yeasts made here in the United States are often so aggressive. No wonder yeast is such a prevalent allergy. The combination of both gluten and yeast would be devastating for me to eat. Both could easily blow out sensitive stomachs for anyone with yeast and fungus challenges.

Now, eating foods that are gluten free is a massive growing segment of our population. Many, except the manufacturers, want to get away from pesticides and genetically modified (GMO) foods. Many foods are modified through nature or humans pairing two seeds together. Pesticides pose a bigger health risk than the naturally occurring GMO foods. However, the GMO foods that have neurotoxic effects are those that were modified with viruses or pesticides. The major challenge is that big food companies are allowed to modify foods, and they are circumventing the FDA and EPA by rinsing the seeds in Roundup pesticide with the active ingredient glyphosate.

---

[10] Subway Wasn't the Only Chain to Use the 'Yoga Mat Chemical' in Its Bread. Published April 8, 2016. Accessed April 11, 2021. https://www.eater.com/2016/8/8/12403338/subway-yoga-mat-chemical-mcdonalds-burger-king-wendys

The rinsing makes the chemical systemic in the food, bringing higher amounts for our stomach to deal with than ever before. Glyphosate is patented as an antibiotic, with tragic effects on our stomach and country.

Today, many of the snack foods we eat are thousands of times more toxic than before. Zach Bush, MD, states in his documentary, Farmer's Footprint, "Our rainwater, especially in Mississippi, comprises of 75% glyphosate. That Mississippi river valley stretch has the highest cancer rate." Our gut is supposed to be strong and absorptive. Glyphosate instantly breaks it apart. Dr. Bush is on a mission to restore our gut and our farming back to organic ways. His product ION*Biome, (IonBiome.com) is one soil-based supplement that can repair the damage. Plants get their nutrients from the soil, and so can we.

Glyphosate, in the herbicide Roundup, is water-soluble. It is in our rain and hence all crops. Thank you, Dr. Bush, for bringing such an amazing product to facilitate rebinding the health of our gut microbiome and the future of farming. A squirt or teaspoon of it in your glass of water will save you and your child's stomach health. When my daughter reads this book, she will now know that I put ION in nearly every glass of water I serve her.

Howard Cohn, DC, created the product Recovery with molecular hydrogen. This essentially puts oxygen and hydrogen back into your system. Oxygen is one of the missing components to wellness, performance, and recovery. I feel like I took an ozone sauna after I take his Recovery supplement.

Bliss Intake.

This knowledge combines over 30 years of my own experience being gluten free and building the energy systems of the body for optimal performance. I include some nutrition portions of other proven programs. *Eat Right for Your Type* will guide you in maximizing learning about your metabolism, hydration, optimal blood type food matching, and food pairing. Much of the food pairing I follow comes from Ori Hofmekler and his book, *The Warrior Diet*, a pioneer in burning fat as fuel. You will learn how to confidently choose high quality protein foods and good fats and whole grains, organic vegetables, and fruits. You will learn to avoid and replace man-made processed foods containing harmful GMO and other allergenic by-products, such as synthetic pesticides, synthetic ingredients, preservatives, hormones, gluten, and anti-nutrients (resistant starch), while enjoying good natural foods, knowing you are nurturing your body and soul with yummy food choices.

The focus of Bliss Intake is to learn what to eat and look for that will allow you to thrive. When the body does not have enough of the proper intake, it can't perform at its peak level. I want you to have boundless energy, digest, and enjoy a lifestyle that revolves around eating to feed your soul. To do so, we will teach you many of the food pairings to burn fat as a primary fuel source and allow you to make healthy, enjoyable lifestyle choices.

By pairing the right foods together, you will avoid the spiking and crashing experienced when relying mostly on carbohydrates, sugars, or caffeine. This feeds the oxidative, glycolytic, and phosphagen energy systems covering your aerobic, anaerobic, and reserve energy systems. This is a food-pairing guide combining proteins, fats, and carbohydrates to create the optimal fuel your body needs to consistently work at its potential. It is one of the most sustainable lifestyle intakes you can find.

Bliss food pairing is a guide to a low processed carbohydrate (man-made baked goods), high green and *good* fat (LCHF) intake. The three main types of food sources that fuel your body are proteins (meats, eggs, and dairy), carbohydrates (grains, fruits, and vegetables), and fats (butters and oils). Your energy is most efficient when good fats and a balance of the above are eaten for your body type. Athleticism.com has a new Palm Kernel MCT oil, Lean Oil, that helps fuel the body with an incredible oil that is 10X better than coconut MCT. You can also find it at LeanOil.com. It gets you ripped and facilitates in massive weight loss.

Common positive changes to expect include weight loss, increased physical strength, energy, mental vigor, sinus pressure relief, and mental clarity. These healthy changes are sustainable, and your body will reward you when you continue to make sound food pairing and exercise choices in your everyday un-diet lifestyle.

Why is the pairing of food so important?

First, your body releases certain enzymes and acids to digest what you eat.

Second, the food you eat and how you pair it together determines your fuel source. We follow the simple concept that sugar spikes and crashes you, while good fat provides sustained energy.

We have a guide that simplifies learning how to fuel your body, to set you up for sustained success eating at every meal, snacking, and enjoying meals out. We are born with microflora, which is the good bacteria in our digestive tract. The body receives a diverse microbiome from eating different sources of greens. There are multiple layers of immune-rich acidophilus, highly beneficial for the body. This is meant to protect the intestinal tract from parasites, bad food, fungi, and prevent pathogens from leaking into the intestinal wall to the blood stream (leaky gut syndrome). This intake program will support your natural defenses. Thanks to Ori's early research, here are several beneficial combinations, which include:[11]

---

[11] Hofmekler O. *The Warrior Diet*. Blue Snake Books; 2007.

- Bacon and eggs
- Beans and eggs
- Steak and eggs
- Beans and rice
- Cauliflower, rice, and cheese
- Fruit and cheese
- Steak and salad (protein and vegetables are good with everything)
- Vegetables and potato
- Nuts and seeds
- Wine and cheese (alcohol with protein, fat, or a vegetable is good)
- Wine and nuts
- Plant Protein and berries* (used as snacks)

When you start to burn fat as your primary fuel source, you will see a reduction in cravings. It does not mean you shouldn't eat fast fuel during competition. It means, overall, you have a more consistent energy source. You will not yearn for that bad food. I went from eating bags of potato chips, to eating a handful of them. You will not have the inconsistent energy, spiking due to low blood sugar and crashing throughout the day. Yes, your body will start to transform, shed the winter coat, decrease inflammation, and you will feel so much better in every way.

Inflammation will show up in a number of ways. If you are allergic or have a sensitivity to a food, it may cause the weight scale to rise or your joints to swell. You can easily feel it in your finger joints the next day. Your skin will react around your lower mouth, or you may even experience canker sores. The glial cells in the brain are important for neurotransmission. Any inflammation or trauma will affect them and your cognitive skills.

The gut is also known as 'the second brain.' Avoiding inflammation, while keeping the immune and digestive systems healthy and strong, is an integral part of gut-brain health. Dr. Michael Gershon wrote a book titled *The Second Brain*, devoting his career to understanding the human bowel (the stomach, esophagus, small intestine, and colon). His over 30 years of research have led to an extraordinary rediscovery: nerve cells in the gut act as a brain. Not only do they act as the brain, they are so similar and have more nerve cells. This is an incredible finding. We now know that, when we feed our stomach with a proper intake and create a rich microbiome, our brain will thrive. This will lead to better decision-making during competition.

Your gut, your second brain, communicates with your actual brain and body through symptoms of digestion, gas, cramps, acne, and aesthetics (you can see if we store food as fat). The biggest symptom I look for is lack of elimination (fecal should be sizable, effortless, occur daily, and look like your colon).

Elimination tells a lot of the story. I had a friend in college that got a hernia from pushing too strong when going to the bathroom. After surgery to fix it, all the doctor said was, "Don't push so hard." He did not advise to change my friend's intake so he could easily eliminate his waste. I had years where my stool looked like rabbit poop. I just had no idea. How clueless are we? I had rabbit poop, gas, stomach pains, bad breath, bumps on the back of my tongue from not digesting food, a flakey scalp, and I carried baby fat for too long. My body was telling me over and over to make a change. I was tough, but I wasn't as aware as I thought I was.

When under immense stress, with no time to catch up, your body will need a natural boost and enzymes to help with absorption. Doing detoxes is highly important. Ozone saunas or foot baths will help clear out heavy metal and toxicity, allowing the good to work even better. Many supplements are designed to not only strengthen your mitochondria, but also to increase the efficiency of energy production and delivery mechanisms. With any fatigued or overheated state, recovery mode, or wanting to build up your reserves, proper supplementation is important.

Here is a simple checklist that would have saved me lots of stomachaches and my friend a hernia. In a nutshell…(pun intended), eat foods with more bioavailable nutrients and a program that entails:

- ✔ Gluten free (avoid wheat, rye, oats, barley (malt), hops, spelt, couscous, khorasan wheat (kamut), semolina, wheat bran, and wheat germ)

- ✔ Eat non-GMO and avoid processed foods, preservatives, hormones, and artificial foods and dyes
- ✔ Avoid synthetic and man-made sugars
- ✔ Eat real, organic whole foods and grass fed (non-GMO grass) when possible…foods that are raised and grown closest to as if they were wild
- ✔ Pair proper foods together
- ✔ Eat quality protein in the morning, ideally after high intensity workouts (approximately 20- to 30-minute workouts, minimum)
- ✔ Sit, chew, and dine at your meals
- ✔ No need to eat a meal if you are not hungry
- ✔ Go out to dinner and enjoy indulging a few times a week
- ✔ Eat grains less frequently and balance animal fats
- ✔ Look at eating foods grown through biodynamics
- ✔ Balance animal fats
- ✔ Eat good fats (grass fed butter, olive oil, avocado, and nuts)
- ✔ Eat a starchy meal once a week for dinner; be diverse
- ✔ Wine and cheese are a good combo (if you drink wine and eat dairy)
- ✔ Eat a variety of cruciferous or brassica vegetables

Naturally sweet foods are more enjoyable, especially when they are real and fresh. Eating the proper fats and oils will buffer the insulin spikes for when you do consume sugar. Use natural sweeteners like honey, syrup, raw sugar, or dates. They may have a higher glycemic index, but are more recognizable to absorb, especially when you have proper insulin buffers like, Lean Oil. Purchase gum made with xylitol. When you need some carbonation, avoid soda or beer and reward yourself with sparkling mineral water instead. Just read the ingredients. When you can follow this balanced intake, you will see your body become more alkaline. By pairing foods to burn fat, you can eat proper amounts with more sustained energy and get quick fuel from the foods that are naturally occurring.

Drink.

There are too many water choices, and most of them are not optimal for performance. So much of our water is riddled with antidepressants, birth control pills, and other pharmaceutical medications people flush down the toilet. People often say that filtered water is best, but there is no way to filter all that stuff. Others claim to drink alkaline water, but although it has a great pH, it does not have minerals for hydration. Find your favorite clean source of mountain or spring water. This spring water is alive with natural minerals.

Look at what the rain does to feed nature to confirm how necessary minerals are for hydration and life. I have a new lemon tree that would not grow very much, even after I added fertilizer and watered it more often. Not until we got hit with above normal winter precipitation did the tree start to take shape. It grew a few feet and the leaves turned greener than ever, yielding a solid crop of the sweetest tasting lemons. I could eat pieces of it like a grapefruit and eat the peel. It was unbelievable what natural rainwater did for the health of this tree. The tree needed minerals to get healthy, and so do we.

There are so many spring and mountain waters to choose from. It is advised to drink multiple sources and avoid the purified water leached of all its minerals. When the water is alive, it will carry more minerals and have a higher alkalinity. Your body is over 70% water, and you want it to flow. Drink at least 8 to 10 glasses per day or half your body weight in ounces. Intuitively, I follow the APO diet recommendation of consuming a lot of water at once. My drinking is more like a camel, so I wake up and drink a few glasses of water, and I continue to drink that amount in about 3-4 servings throughout the day. This is achievable, and you will see less fatigue with proper hydration. If you are used to drinking sugary drinks and need flavor, just add lemon or lime. A glass of lemon water first thing in the morning is one of the best things you can do for your alkaline health.

One of the biggest trends you will see in the US in the next decade is drinking deuterium-depleted water. Deuterium is a heavier and larger isotope of hydrogen. The less deuterium in the water, the better it is for your health. They call it light water.

Dehydration is a stressor on the body. Any other water than spring water will provide little value whatsoever. This will lead to fatigue, muscle weakness, and muscle tightness. Any adrenal challenges need to hydrate more. Stating the obvious, anyone dealing with toxicity should drink more water to flush the toxins.

Here are 3 ways to tell when you are dehydrated.

1. There will be very little saliva in your mouth. When you speak your lips will tend to stick and smack together. This is also called cotton mouth. You will get a dry, frothy feeling and see white formation on each side of your mouth.
2. You get tired in the early afternoon. I have too many clients who have afternoon fatigue, and all they need to combat is to change their water to mountain spring water and drink more water.
3. Look at your skin and compare it to others' skin. The people who look like they have snakeskin, with a very dry, wrinkly texture, have had a lifetime of dehydration.

There are lots of trendy water places popping up. As cool as they look and as hip as their bottles are, their water is mostly clean, dead water, with very little hydration value. Mountain spring water hydrates you better. Muscle testing shows your body is weak with dead water and strong with spring water. Our body needs those natural minerals to thrive. Supplementing with trace minerals is helpful, but I'm all about starting with the right source.

Once you have the clean water, run it through a LoveItWater.com system. It creates the structured, linear water molecules to have more viscous and absorption properties. Dave Jensen, DC, believes this is the ultimate hydration for us. This proper hydration is the key to wellness and performance.

Avoid sports drinks and sodas as they have too much artificial sugar and artificial everything. The FDA labels artificial colors and flavors because they are so detrimental to our health. Drink sparkling mineral water when you want a cold, carbonated drink. Consume carbonated drinks in moderation as the carbonation can leach your body of minerals. If you want apple, grapefruit, or cranberry juice, make sure there is no added sugar. Just make it as close to natural as possible. Also, if you are constantly craving juices, dilute your juice 50/50 with water. You will still get your fix without the vast amount of sugar. Hot or cold green tea can have endless medicinal benefits.

If coffee or green tea is your thing, enjoy drinking a cup or two per day of unsweetened coffee or green tea. When making soup or other goods that require water, use spring water. I have had bone broth that flipped my stomach due to the poor-quality tap water used. Even if you boil it, the heavy metals will still find a sensitive stomach.

Just to give you a heads up, when you put pure minerals in distilled water, the water will become the purest form of mineral water. The distilled water will ignite the mineral properties.

Chapter 3: Nerve Health, Stress & Stressors.

Most industry experts and doctors focus on working or treating the muscles and bones. My focus is working with the nerves. I not only fast-twitch train the system with speed work, but I also work with primal reflexes and nerve restoration. I feel the nerves supersede all others most of the time. A primary effort when treating clients is to stabilize an individual faster than ever, through nerve restoration. Once treated, I typically average getting about 20% more strength instantly. I can easily quantify it on an ARX machine. My prediction is that treating the nervous system will become one of the biggest areas of focus in the next decade. Nerves travel 325 mph through the body. When I can dial the nerve speed all the way up, the results are remarkable. Muscle testing shows the level of responsiveness and the level of nerve health. The muscle sends a message to the myotomes at light speed. From here, we get a strong or delayed muscle and nerve response. After the treatment, the results are instantaneous, and any delay will now become instantly strong. You can say goodbye to the pain when the underlying issue is not a major structural challenge.

My day-to-day work revolves around treating individuals to get them stronger, more flexible, preventing injuries and facilitating getting people out of an injury state through primal and motor nerve work. The sensory nerve work can improve audio and visual processing, helping with your spatial awareness and court/field presence. The sensory nerve protocol also doubles as our concussion protocol in helping reconnect brain pathways that were disrupted from the trauma. Here is the short list of what I do when treating:

- Nerve rehabilitation (cranial, cervical, and lumbar nerves)
- Nerve restoration (sensory and motor nerves)
- Primal Pain Reflex Release Technique (PRRT) joint stability
- Active isolated stretching
- Posture
- Lymph flushes
- Emotional clearings
- Ambidexterity development
- Balance
- Sound therapy
- Light therapy

The central nervous system (CNS) has always been a focal point of my athletic development. The CNS includes the brain and spine. It controls all activities of the body, including thought, movement, and provides sensation (light touch, deep touch, etc.). The peripheral nerves connect to the CNS outside of it communicating to muscles.

The techniques I use are a direct and effective way to communicate with the vagus nerve and dura mater. I teach my certification courses and seminars on how to do both a manual nerve technique and light therapy. Others using light therapy flood the body with light, hoping the injured area gets energized. That is very helpful, but proper techniques get even faster results. The treatments I use also spark the body's endogenous opioid receptors[12]. This is just another added benefit to feeling better, resulting in performing stronger and faster.

The process of improving nerve responsiveness or stability is also used for developing bilateral sensory sports performance. As you will see, with all the Whole Brain exercises we do, our progressions will entail doing several coordination movements, coupled with ambidexterity development, all at once. This stresses the brain, accordingly, allowing the brain entrainment and plasticity to improve. This is the essence of ATHLETICISM. Develop coordination and ambidexterity while stressing multiple systems. A simple Neuro Stacking example is balancing on a BOSU ball while juggling and doing math equations.

I currently work with a USA gold medalist. She is vying for another spot and gold medal on the 2020 USA Women's Water Polo Team. During her double days, they work out about 6 hours per day. In order to keep her fresh, I have to do nerve restoration. Once the nerves reconnect, they can heal faster, allowing her to stay at the top of her game without neuro fatigue. We have every recovery mechanism

---

[12] How does the opioid system control pain, reward, and addictive behavior? Published October 15, 2007. Accessed April 11, 2021. https://www.sciencedaily.com/releases/2007/10/071014163647.htm

going for her. We even make sure her sleep is optimized, and she can wear an IntelliSkin posture shirt when sleeping. Lance Armstrong used to use this similar type of nerve work. Although he took steroids, he still had the best recovery systems that were just as extensive as ours. These nerve treatments are also amazing for healing injuries and getting clients out of a pain state.

I recently treated a 15-year veteran and former NFL player. I used primal reflex release techniques along with nerve restoration techniques. His neck was in pain, so I used nerve work and Neuro Stacking to get him over 80% better in about 10 minutes. Feeling 80% better is the average result our clients see from this nerve work. If you are not addressing your nerves, your performance will be limited, and injuries will not go away as fast as they should.

One of the best analogies of nerve health and nerve strength versus nerve fatigue is watching the Major League Baseball World Series. The pitchers must throw as hard as they can multiple nights and sometimes with only one night's rest. You can see the neuro fatigue in their throwing arms. They will miss their spots, and the hitters can easily see the pitches. With more men on base or home runs, they will rotate to the next pitcher who will, more often than not, have a similar neuro fatigue and outcome. A quick ATHLETICISM Neuro Stacking treatment could refresh their arm instantly and improve performance.

Light treatments are restorative as well. Just as plants garner energy through light at the cellular level, so do we. I use near-infrared and a pulsed red, low frequency LED to restore nerve connectivity to the motor and sensory nerves. I can upregulate the cranial, cervical, and lumbar nerves to improve performance. Light therapy is one of the oldest therapies. What does the medical world do when babies are born with jaundice? They flood them with light.

As a whole, our civilization has gotten away from just sitting in front of a fire absorbing the heat, light, and sound. We don't hear much about people traveling to the Swiss Alps for heliotherapy clinics from worry about the ultraviolet rays. The concept of targeted light therapy I do is now a specific art to rid the body of pain, stabilize, increase range of motion, and improve performance. My beautiful and genius wife touts me as being one of the biggest trendsetters in the health industry. She hypes me as the earliest in the gluten free movement, as well as one of the first to use BOSU balls, kettlebells, ozone therapy, IV drips, foot baths, cup stacking, light therapy, frequency healing with our Grounding Bags, having EMF awareness, Qi Gong, stretching therapy, sound therapy and now, doing nerve work for sports performance.

The question I get asked most frequently is, "How long does that stability last?" This brings us to why I am sharing my daily treatments with you. This book details stressors and how to avoid them. Once we establish a strong nerve connection, the nerve strength holds until there is a massive trauma or stressor. However, there are often multiple layers to peel and strengthen. I have identified 3 ways to downregulate the connection. I briefly touched on the stressors mentioned earlier in the book. The 3 major ways that your body shuts down these connections include:

1. Emotional (stress, thoughts, feelings, or emotions)
2. Structural and Physical (too little work, too much work, or a trauma)
3. Biochemical (bad food, drink, environment, or EMF)

Many call this the triad of health. In my practice, I make sure this triad is properly addressed or my work will take longer than needed. Once the health and intake are in order, and the stressors are eliminated or minimized, the focus can move to developing the body and using this work as an enhancer and another way to develop the nervous system.

Optimal health is a balance of all systems. Many of the major systems include:

- Nervous system
- Musculoskeletal system
- Circulatory system
- Digestive system
- Endocrine system
- Immune system
- Lymphatic system
- Reproductive system
- Electromagnetic system

When I work with clients to get rid of their pain or injuries, I look at the whole body starting with the nerves and primal emotional holding patterns. There are easy ways to see what is wrong through muscle testing. When there is adrenal fatigue, the sartorius muscle will test weak. I evaluate and fix the underlying challenge(s). So many just look at the symptoms and treat them. Finding the cause is the more aware approach. The cause could be a lack of good water, weak hips, poor posture, arches of the foot collapsing, your electric car…the list can feel endless. Even a concussion can blow out your hormone levels and gut. I often draw from all my various trainings to solve these challenges. Many of the chemical balances rely on a proper intake, detoxing, ridding stressors, and supplementing with vitamins and minerals. This is why I have dedicated a big section of the book to intake.

To get the nerve treatment to hold for longer periods, I have to stack the treatments. Essentially, I test the eyes down to the toes, all at the same time. Whether we are developing multiple systems at once or treating multiple parts of one system, Athleticism Neuro Stacking is essential for performance.

·································

Emotional thoughts, feelings, and stress are pretty self-explanatory. If you are worried about family, friends, money, work, or relationships, those are all emotional stressors. In Oriental medicine, the elements fire, earth, metal, water, and wood all correlate to specific organs. Each has a list of emotions that are attached to them. The body does not know the difference between past, present, and future. This is known as epigenetics. Until the conscious mind meets the subconscious, a limiting emotional holding patterns exists, keeping you in a sympathetic nervous system, in fight or flight mode. Dr. Bruce Lipton found that we can kill every part of the cell, but it's not until the protein receptors are killed that the cell dies, and we can return to the parasympathetic mode. Releasing these holding patterns can now change the genetic predisposition to certain conditions. This is incredible research by Dr. Lipton. The LifeLine Technique is a system that can bring Dr. Lipton's work into reality.

We end up holding on to a lot of emotions. Not until the conscious meets the subconscious will we release these holding patterns. This is why I do emotional clearings through The LifeLine Technique. This is the way to access the power centers as Dr. Darren Weissman calls them. "The super-conscious (thoughts, feelings, and beliefs) all connect to the collective conscious." You don't have to be a doctor to clear the protein receptors that store the emotions. As I mentioned earlier in the book, just give the sign language hand gesture for love and say, "Infinite love and gratitude." This will help you heal, recover, create, and not give your power away during competition.

Biochemical stressors are:

1. Food
2. Drink
3. Air
4. EMF

We have already covered most of these. Even food or drinks that are inflammatory nightshade foods or those you are allergic to are stressors. Heavy metals are another big biochemical stressor that can come from our air, food, tap water, Novocaine, metal fillings in teeth, metal plates mending a broken bone, vaccinations, and can even be passed on from our parents, as Dr. Pompa states. Andrew Pallos, DDS, shares on my GoBeyondSummit.com that the only legal place to put mercury is in our mouth. We can't put mercury in our landfills, but we can put it in our mouths and vaccinations…. Explain that?!

Human biology is an important part to understand for our health. Please know that current viral studies show a virus is a dead protein that does not eat, produce energy, or reproduce. When we are introduced to a toxin or toxic environment, we produce a virus or dead protein as our own way to adapt and flush. Our Adaptive Immune Response balances out our body as we upgrade and adapt to the new environment. Our bodies and the planet are built on viruses, bacteria, and fungi. Zach Bush, MD, states, "There are 10^{31} viruses in the air, that is 31 zeros after a 1. There is about that same amount in the water, our bodies, and soil." These viruses are self-limiting, meaning they are not meant to kill or we would not be here for billions of years. The message here is that contagions are atmospheric and everywhere. Clearing the stressors, flushing your body, and building your gut microbiome are the main elements to health and wellness. Look to yourself to heal. Wearing a mask, distancing from others, or taking a drug/vaccine with nanotechnology to make you a GMO human is not health and wellness.

An electromagnetic field (EMF), better known as radiation, is a massive challenge for our body to process. Why? Because it de-charges your body, small intestines, teeth, and eyes. These EMFs are the current #1 constant stressor on our body, being a gateway to injury and illness. Less oxygen is supplied, thus, affecting your low brain wave state during performance. Hertz measures cycles per second or wave frequency = cycles. Amplitude is wave height = intensity. Humans optimize at a very low brain wave state compared to billions of waves/second from man-made radio frequency. EMFs come in 3 forms: electricity, dirty electricity, and radio frequency. Electricity wired into your home or any outlet and appliance is measured in milligauss (mG). Dirty electricity is the sparking in the power lines from bad wiring, dimmer switches, rats eating wires, and solar panel batteries. Radio frequency (RF) is any wireless signal. The RF signal strengths are only getting stronger and are growing at rapid speed. Brussels, Belgium, is the first major city to ban 5G, and I am certain many more places will. Countries like France banned

Wi-Fi in elementary schools years ago to protect the young brains and their developing reproductive organs.

Dr. Michael Gooing in Costa Mesa, California, understands the strength of EMFs and can treat these challenges. When you are aware and get the stressors out, you can detox, heal, and perform. Dr. Gooing breaks it down like this…

"1 DIGITAL X-RAY = 30 OLD FILM X-RAYS

3G = 800 X-RAYS OVER 24 HOURS

4G = 1600 X-RAYS OVER 24 HOURS

5G = 100 X 4G

MERCURY = 2 X 5G

SAN ONOFRE NUCLEAR = 20 X 5G

4G/5G/SAN ONOFRE/SMART METERS CUMULATIVE = 50 X 5G"

Why is wireless RF so challenging for us? The speed of the wave is 10 zeros faster than how we sleep, recover, perform, and optimize. Plus, the waves are polarizing and meant to go in one direction. We are used to the sun's waves that are unpolarized and distribute equally in every direction. The current 4G Wi-Fi is up to speeds of approximately 20 billion waves per second. 5G is nonstop, at 60 to 90 billion waves per second, similar to microwave weaponry levels. All for faster Internet with zero regard for the environment or your health. EMF stressors affect your deep sleep, disrupting melatonin production, neurotransmitter, and nucleotide (stem cell) production. This lack of deep sleep, pineal gland disruption, and a decharged body, become a gateway for injury or disease. Any heavy metal in the body will also be charged by the EMF, so it is important to do detoxes of heavy metals and amalgams.

How does EMF become a gateway, you ask? The constant vibration opens the voltage-gated calcium channels (VGCC), letting positive calcium into a negative cell. This excess calcium leads to most major health challenges, says Dr. Martin Pall.[13] Man-made EMF has a positive charge, while the earth, ocean, and humans have a negative charge.

When we rid, repel, or ground the EMF stressors, we will stay in a deeper sleep state. All routers, cell phones, and smart meters send out billions of waves per second. Our brain attempts to figure out what those signals are. We then wake up and often stay in more of a twilight sleep, not getting a full night of rest. Turn those wireless signals off at night.

The pineal gland, often referred to as your third eye, is responsible for producing melatonin. I am big on making sure your glands are functioning, so your sleep is not impaired.

---

[13] Pall ML. Electromagnetic fields act via activation of voltage-gated calcium channels to produce beneficial or adverse effects. *J Cell Mol Med*. 2013;17(8):958-965.

The thymus can also crash with 5G, ultimately throwing off your entire energy systems. An uninterrupted circadian rhythm in sleep is so important to your hormone production and recovery.

I have clients who lived with excessively high electricity exposure of mG in their home for over a decade. The wife was a former pro athlete, aged 44, and got early menopause. The son, aged 12, ate as healthily as possible and got diabetes. When I shared the dangers of EMF, they instantly made major changes. They moved away from the electricity source to the beach. More sunlight and grounding from the earth and ocean shifted their energy instantly. They rewired their new home to have the lowest possible EMF levels. They purchased my EMFRocks.com Grounding Bags to repel and ground the invisible EMF. I gave them my specific EMF detox protocol. Within a few months, all symptoms normalized faster and better than their doctor had ever seen. The sunlight, earthing in the sand, unplugging routers at night, repelling, and grounding got them back closer to the Schumann Resonance (about 7.83 Hz) healthy range so they could heal and thrive.

Our Grounding Bag on EMFRocks.com is one of the best products I have ever seen. It contains special colloid, Tesla rocks for repelling and grounding, creating a faraday effect around your body. Put it near yourself, and it helps heal injuries and recharge your body. Several bags (3 to 6) will ground an entire 2,000sf home, and one in or under each bed, for the best night's sleep. With our deep sleep state and the earth at such a low frequency, eliminating EMF from the bedroom and getting Grounding Bags is huge for performance. This is frequency healing at its best, like walking barefoot in a bag. The more healing frequencies around us, the more we can sleep, heal, and amplify our frequency for health and performance.

The physical stressors are easy to grasp. Doing too little, too much, or experiencing a trauma can change the nerve strength. When the body receives a trauma, bruise, strain, sprain, or fracture, the nerves most likely will have a delayed response. The swelling will protect and start to mend the joint or muscle, but re-establishing the nerve connections is not normally the focus of healing. Over-trained and under-recovered nerve connections will muscle test with a delayed response. This delay or neuro fatigue is when injuries occur. The delay will directly show the lack of speed of the reflexes and limit true performance.

Now you may have awareness in more areas then you imagined. Awareness of clearing the stressors will improve performance without doing anything else. When you add in the rest of our program, your performance just keeps getting better. We now continue this journey of awareness and creativity in Whole Body exercises to elevate your performance.

ATHLETICISM

Part II. Whole Body Coordination.

Chapter 4: Whole Body Exercises.

When we challenge your coordination and teach you to move efficiently and balanced, it will expand your body and brain plasticity. The fast-twitch fibers will come alive. You will find a rhythm that will make you faster, more powerful, and better than ever.

When I first read about Dean Brittenham making athletes better athletes, I was blown away by his ability to make them faster and jump higher. I was looking for a run, jump, or speed and power program, but I didn't realize it until I saw it. The concept was amazing, and the drills were incredible. The subtle cues were life changing for me. When I was able to do my first workout with Dean, it was one of the best experiences of my life. The entire concept of having a balance, joint stability, stretching, and eye-hand ambidexterity warm-up was revolutionary. Then, to go outside on a track and learn how to move for the first time in my life was surreal. To compare my coordination with kids and pros in the same class was one of the most fun experiences ever. I now had a coach who made working out fun, while challenging my coordination at the same time. It was me versus my own coordination and gravity, compared to a coach yelling to run faster. After years of searching, I had finally found the most robust performance program. I also found my passion in life.

Doing speed and coordination drills is where it all comes together. It doesn't matter if you are on a field, court, track, park, or street. This is where the magic happens. This is where you get moving, seeing and feeling the difference in your speed. It is where we begin to challenge your coordination, then speed, and then power. This is where we humble the best athletes in the world. This is where younger athletes develop coordination and more. We will see how much rhythm you have and how light you are on your feet. We will teach you how to run, skip, bound, shuffle, and change directions. We will get you firing equally off each foot, accelerating and decelerating. You will learn plyometrics with little and big jumps. This is where you learn footwork and how to be light, nimble, fast, and powerful. This is where you develop explosive coordination and add a new dimension to your game. If I had to say go do one thing from this book, I would have to say, "Do our speed and coordination Whole Body exercises, and you will exponentially improve your performance."

Who are the fastest athletes? Answer: track and field athletes.

Dean Brittenham was a strength coach and track and field coach. He knew how to teach athletes how to run and run fast. This ATHLETICISM Whole Body program began as a track-based program. We use all the basic drills that the fastest athletes in the world use. We do these drills with more awareness, coordination, rhythm, and non-linear movement so every different athlete will benefit. We know how to strengthen your feet, toes, every joint, and the prime movers in the body to optimize speed. We use the most effective stretching systems that get rapid results. We follow the scientific formulas for speed and power. This is actual science, not some new drill that looks cool. You will learn efficiency of movement for every movement system.

I didn't know how to juggle or dunk a basketball. I didn't know how to skip or that there are numerous ways to skip. I didn't even know how to run. I didn't know what part of the foot to run on. I didn't know bounding made you faster. I didn't know how to shuffle and move laterally. Doing years of tennis and moving laterally across the base line, I didn't know that doing heel-toe movements at certain times was slowing me down. I didn't know how to use an efficient first step. There were endless cues that I could not believe I missed from all the coaching and my own lack of awareness. This program is exactly what I had been searching for.

By the time I was 18, there were not many kids who logged more time on a soccer field or tennis court than I did. I had some excellent coaches and I had never seen anything remotely close to what Dean taught. All my drills with other coaches were done in straight lines for fitness. No one moved in semicircles or figure 8's. No one spoke of eccentric change of direction power. These concepts were decades ahead of their time. I knew I felt and performed amazingly after. To validate it further, Dean had proved the program repeatedly with professional athletes and teams in most major sports.

Niednagel is on record saying that, "Jim Courier, the former #1 Tennis player in the world, was one of the biggest overachieving brain types." Jim was working with Dean at the time he jumped from the top 25 to top 5 in the world. This is a massive example of how Whole Body Whole Brain development and Neuro Stacking improves performance. This is a significant validation for our ATHLETICISM programs. We have unlimited success stories from all our years of athletic development.

> Niednagel is on record saying that,
> **Jim Courier, the former #1 Tennis player in the world, was one of the biggest overachieving brain types.**
> Jim was working with Dean at the time he jumped from the top 25 to top 5 in the world.

John Mallinger, a PGA golfer, jumped up 90 spots on the tour in one year working with me and doing Whole Body Whole Brain development. John Cook won 9 of his PGA Champion Tour victories training with me and our ATHLETICISM programs. He finished 5th, 4th, and 3rd in the Charles Schwab Cup Championship. Matt Fuerbringer also finished as high as #2 with 8 professional wins on the AVP pro beach volleyball tour. His name is on the Manhattan Beach pier, with our ATHLETICISM logo tattooed on his shoulder. Adrian Gonzalez was the MLB's first overall pick in the draft and one of the most successful MLB players. It works for high school athletes, too. The list goes on.

That emphasis of developing a Whole Body with more pathways from the brain to the body through non-linear coordination movements is one of our secrets in athletic and human performance development. It complements all your coach's efforts. You will be able to do what your sports coach wants easier than before. Implementing these similar concepts and exercises, I will show you how to develop these connections at an early age or as soon as you begin. Many of our ATHLETICISM Whole Body program components consist of:

- Figure 8's and non-linear movements
- Rhythmic movements
- Cross-crawl movements
- Coordination movements
- Speed and power development
- Neuro Stacking of multiple exercises
- Balance
- Nerve health
- Joint stability
- Light therapy
- Sound therapy
- Eye development
- Hand/foot dexterity

There are virtually unlimited ways to tap into developing more pathways from the brain to the body, but we have figured out special recipes. Remember, teaching an individual to be ambidextrous does not take the one-side dominance away; it makes the whole stronger, getting rid of the weak links. Athletes must be just as explosive off their right foot and left foot, no matter their dominant side. If you believe you are only as strong as your weakest link, why wouldn't we get rid the weak links? These links apply to strength, flexibility, coordination, and eye and brain development. ATHLETICISM is one of the few performance programs in the country to actually have a non-linear movement ambidexterity program. Keep in mind, all the greatness happens in the details of every exercise and modality. We have incorporated several of our techniques and the specific tips below for you to follow, build upon, and benefit.

The body has a specific energy system and flow to it. Sprinters run opposite arm, opposite leg, right?! This is a cross-crawl pattern that is innate in our energy flow. When healthy babies learn to move, you will see them move in an opposite arm, opposite leg cross-crawling motion. Crawling is a massive developmental stage of the body. Pavel Kolar brought it to our attention. There are specific developmental movement stages that kids must go through. We use these cross-crawl patterns when moving in every direction.

The more fun and engaged they are, the higher the benefits. When activities are pleasurable and done in a semicircle or figure 8, the biggest hormonal lifts of dopamine occur via the basal ganglia, known as the reward circuit. Your energy frequencies become optimized. No matter the exercise, challenging the body's coordination will develop more pathways and improved performance. Simple coordination exercises take people out of their comfort zone, are fun, challenging, and will improve their body and brain plasticity. The key is to find the weak links and challenge them progressively, developing more coordination and speed. With these methods, the results are incredible.

This is not some workout to make you puke. It is not a boot camp! This is not a workout from a guy who has a certification that does straight-line ladder drills and box jumps, claiming he is a performance guy. This is an anaerobic system with intelligence where you rest between sets. Even our barriers are soft foam, so if you step on them, they give, and you won't get injured. This is the most thoughtful, aware performance program.

Athletic development for the body means establishing more connections from your eyes and brain to your body. Doing just one sport repeatedly does not get you to master your ATHLETICISM Whole Body Whole Brain. It often limits you, trains you in one dimension, and sets you up for burnout or potentially developing an overuse injury. When you must groove in a swing with repetitive motions, this extra coordination we teach will only be an enhancer for you.

The progression of the program is also incredible. We start with coordination movements. We increase the speed and intensity as you develop. Then we lengthen the course. Next, we develop power. Wow, it is so simple, yet so effective.

Essentially, this method can also be called developing more coordination, ambidexterity, and cross-crawl rhythm. Whole Body development strengthens the connective symmetry and connection between all quadrants of your brain, vestibular system, to the proprioceptor end points of your body. We are building brain plasticity, so you see, feel, and hear with the road map to go beyond by connecting multiple systems, engaging and adapting to increases of a stimulus. We also change the terrain of your workout. You can start on the surface of your sport, but to help your body adapt, you should train on grass, asphalt, wood courts, hills, and in sand. This is a new paradigm and path for athletic transformation.

Methods & Intangibles.

So much of what I speak about seems to be the intangibles. But, if you saw someone run same arm, same leg, you would notice it, right? This is what I mean by being tangible. When trained, you can see what is right vs. wrong or coordinated vs. uncoordinated. When you actually do the drills, you will see and feel the effects, and they become clearly tangible. ATHLETICISM allows a quality of the following skills relished by observers and competitors alike:

- Explosive coordination
- Vigor
- Grace
- Concentration
- Execution

There is not just one method of exercise that makes an individual better, so I have combined all the major developmental areas with exercises to provide you a comprehensive performance program.

One of the great qualities of developing an individual with our Whole Body method is that it is non-sport and non-activity specific. This means that when you develop speed (fast-twitch muscle fibers), power, balance, eye speed, coordination, and awareness, it transfers directly over into any sport or activity. We can train individuals of all sports, activities, ages, and levels garnering incredible results. Understanding movements, biomechanics, and skill sets of most sports is important to communicate why and how that skill is applicable to the athlete. I will show even more on how the figure 8 movement system applies to most sports. Learning it will improve performance and decrease the risk of injuries.

This method complements the work of a sports coach and allows your coach to be so much more productive and efficient with the team or individual. This development will make individuals more functionally stable, flexible, coordinated, and sound. There is a certain endorphin release that takes place from our entire program collectively. The program results include improving the individual's and team's performance, increasing synergy, confidence, nerve health, and reducing the risk of injuries.

It is so fun to see an entire team gel at the same time from this method. The Pepperdine Men's Tennis team went from #19 to #4 in the nation with our Whole Body Whole Brain development. All the parts must fit. Peter Smith's coaching was incredible, and he brought the fun factor everywhere. Plus, we had the NCAA D1 #1 ranked tennis player, Al Garland, on the team. The synergy we developed was incredible, with many amazing young adults on that team. His team gave it their all, challenged their coordination, and found their flow. They were one of my favorite teams I have ever trained. Peter Smith was hired by USC after that successful season and was one of their most successful head coaches for 17 seasons.

I ran tennis footwork camps with Peter Smith at Pepperdine for a few summers prior. We had great synergy, and he knew he had to bring this program to his team. Back then in the early 2000s, much of the strength staff was limited. Even today, universities do their best but miss on this basic concept of ATHLETICISM's Whole Body Whole Brain. There are a lot of strength coaches with amazing degrees but weak programs. In the last USC strength and conditioning clinic I attended, all the speed and coordination drills were done in straight lines. Many of the NFL players also do straight-line warm-ups. So do many of the MLB and NBA teams and most others. I hope they pick up this book or someone turns them on to it and they connect these rhythms and figure 8's in their warm-ups and workouts.

Picture this for team barrier and speed drill warm-ups: You have 20 athletes. You put 10 on each side. The barriers are set up in semicircles that look like this: ( ).

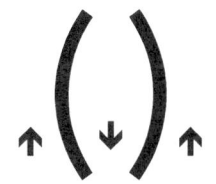

↑ (↓) ↑

The course is done in a figure 8, working on the left semicircle and coming back through the center, then working up on the other semicircle and back through the center. This creates a movement from one side to the other in the shape of a figure 8. The athletes first do speed and coordination drills. The work area is on outside of the semicircles. You rest when you come back through the middle of the course and while you wait your turn to go on the opposite side. Make sure to switch lines and do the same drill on the other side. Again, work on the outside and rest through the center. You build the speed and intensity as you progress. When moving laterally, always face the middle of the course so you work both sides.

This is speed and power interval training at its best. The high intensity, up and down, through the full range of motion is something that is rarely done. It exposes any weak links and develops proper coordination, so when you accelerate forward, you can seamlessly push equally off each side with more dynamic explosiveness. This is also great because you can have various ages and levels of speed, working out in the same line. Since everyone is going up and down fast, barely moving forward, no one will get run over by the big, fast guy. I can work out 20 people easily with this system, as they continue from one drill to the next and get enough rest waiting for the others to finish. The semicircles can be about 10 to 15 yards long, depending on how much you want to spread it out and the size of the group. Only 1 or 2 people are very easy to work out and may require a shorter course or just a few more seconds rest before starting each side. Once you run through our menu of drills and reach the last drill, everyone sprints out of the end of the second semicircle. This transfers the up and down speed, to top-end explosive speed. This is how all individuals and teams should work out. Can you see how the lines flow in a figure 8? We will cover the menu of speed drills later in this book.

When setting up a course at a park or beach, I am always on the lookout for gradual hills and level straightaways for some intrinsic creativity. When we get more sport specific with athletes or teams, it is so fun to set up the workout course on their court or field. For a tennis or volleyball court, we will use half the court, and I will set up the barriers in a figure 8 pattern, outside the lines of the court. This is a bigger than normal training area with more efficient steps. They will learn to cover more of the court efficiently, making the court seem smaller. The goal is having more confidence and being able to cover the court effortlessly.

This coordination program will empower more awareness of the body, efficiently teaching an athlete or team how to find their rhythm for competition. Implement this into your approach of athletic development, day in and out. Get specific on the details.

Use this same semicircle flow during warm-ups prior to competition. Your warm-up becomes a mini workout to prepare your body for competition. When you use it as a warm-up just before your competition, you will not exert as much energy as an actual full workout. You get to full speed up and down on each semicircle, but only for a few reps. Your body needs to be ready to move full speed the second you start your game but not be fatigued at all. You can take an early lead against those opponents who are not fully ready and warmed up. This program wakes up your nervous system, releasing those endorphins, getting you in an amazing rhythm for a massive competitive advantage. I am all about preparing for what you do, establishing a foundation, and having a pre-activity warm-up routine.

Proper biomechanics are crucial for performance. ACSM states, "Biomechanics can be used to maximize the benefits of physical performance in sport, work, and activities of daily living."[14] This is why I will emphasize all the proper mechanics for the major movement systems. Get ready to become very efficient at moving in every direction, even defying gravity.

Building A Solid Foundation.

The first objective is to build a foundation, no matter what level an individual comes to us. A large percentage of my clients are doing physical therapy bridge work with me. This means bridging the gap from when they are discharged from physical therapy (PT) or have a minor injury, not needing PT, to back to their sport better than before. I am bridging the gap between foundation and performance to achieve stability, pain free, full function, better than they were before they were injured. Everyone will win and get amazing results by starting with foundation protocols of stabilizing and lengthening. We all check our egos at the door. Over-lifting or working out past their alkalizing buffers on day one is not going to happen at ATHLETICISM. I am guaranteed to lose a client if they get injured on the first day, even if they are asking for "more" and the doctor said they are allowed to do more. Just slow it down and refocus on the foundations. 10 sets of 10 reps of front squats. 10X10 of overhead squats. Work toward light weight with volume. It may take a bit

---

[14] Battista RA, ed. *ACSM's Resources for the Personal Trainer*, 5e. Philadelphia, PA: Wolters Kluwer; 2018.

longer, but you will not be as likely to get injured, you will make significant gains, and you will love the process. On the flip side, you will thrive and have longevity being active. Often, for professional athletes, it will prolong careers.

Balance, posture, core, proper squatting, coordination, and lung techniques are developed for 2 to 3 months. Any additional weight added to your own body weight will be light. Depending on the lift, start at 1 pound in each hand, and progress from there. Most don't even have the strength to do exercises through a full range with their own body weight, so we slowly progress with volume of body weight movements. Use the proper anatomical cues of shoulders, hips, knee, and second toe are stacked prior to squatting or lifting. Make sure your feet and toes are lined up in a straight line.

Abdominal support with proper breathing is important for overall connectivity. Breathe down to the lowest part of your abdomen and continue the breath around the hips to broaden the foundational support. Most people suck the air in and up into their chest which narrows the core. This chest breathing is considered more of a stress breath. Learning to breath down and around the body takes time. Once developed, your lumbo-pelvic area becomes broader and more stable than ever. This type of breath will be the new bracing system for your back and whole body when lifting.

Make sure to train both sides equally. This includes right to left and front to back. Exercising to be ambidextrous is such an important component in foundation performance development. It will balance out your body, decreasing the risk of injuries.

Whole Brain exercises can also be done during the rest/recovery periods. This will help the individuals stay captivated and challenged during the strength development. Why sit and rest, when you can stand and actively recover, making gains in other areas?

Lateral stability is one of the biggest components for athletes in change of direction and ACL injury prevention. Properly done joint stability will transfer into lateral stability. Ankle weights are great for lateral stability. Just doing straight leg lifts and lateral leg lifts, the knee will become more laterally stable. I have a machine called The Rotator. It strengthens the hips and knees in rotational movements. Most strength protocols only account for flexion and extension, but the knee has a rotational component to it that must be strengthened.

There are 4 movements of the knee or tibiofemoral joint:

1. Flexion
2. Extension
3. Medial rotation of flexed knee
4. Lateral rotation of flexed knee

ATHLETICISM

There are 8 muscles used during flexion and 4 in extension. Medial rotation of a flexed knee uses these five:[15]

1. Semitendinosus
2. Semimembranosus
3. Gracilis
4. Sartorius
5. Popliteus

While lateral rotation of a flexed knee only uses one:

1. Biceps femoris

These are essential to train an athlete for performance and injury prevention. I normally see post-physical therapy clients, but sometimes the clients are not happy with the conventional process of PT. They want a newer approach to healing, faster results, and a better quality of life throughout the healing process. I have a new client who came to me directly out of surgery. She went to her 3-week post operation checkup after her third ACL reconstructive knee surgery. Her surgery was so complex that she had to separate her meniscus surgery, having it a few months prior to the ACL. Plus, they used a quadriceps graft, rarely used. She was supposed to have at least 90° of flexion at this appointment. She was at 125° after the nerve work, stretching, and stability work. Yes, she was 35° ahead of schedule, 3 weeks post-op. So, for the next 4 months, her quality of life became that much better. This foundation work was part of her

---

[15] Biel AR. *Trail Guide to the Body*, 3e. Boulder, CO: Books of Discovery; 2005.

healing process. I only spend 20 minutes with clients, but the results far surpass conventional, or some would call them, antiquated protocols.

You will see the progression within our protocols. You do little jumps before big ones. You develop foundational strength with progression. You do more volume with less weight. All these are common sense. It does not matter what exercise; building a foundation with progression is what we do.

Breathing.

Your breath and performance are directly correlated. First, I teach learning to nasal breath. When you can learn to breathe in through your nose and out through your mouth, your performance will improve, creating a cascade effect. The oxygen floods your body with nitric oxide and the reciprocal positive affect. Dr. Zach Bush will validate that, "This facilitates with the circulation of nutrients for the brain. The Vagal nerve will calm you, and you will get a fuller breath from the bottom of your lungs. The heart rate will correct and potentially decrease 5-10 beats per minute, versus a stress chest breath. Your respiratory system will become more efficient." When doing our speed drills, find a rhythm with your breath.

Learning to breathe in a variety of different ways will exponentially improve your headspace, movement, strength, and endurance. There are many ways to breathe. I will walk through a few breathing sequences to optimize your performance. The 4 sequences I will highlight help with core stability, posture, and energy.

Pavel Kolar shows there is more stability for individuals as they widen and broaden their core. He teaches you to breathe down as low as possible into the lower dantian (several finger spaces below your belly button) and draw the breath around you. This would simulate inflating a pool floatie around your waist. Broaden your core and waist that can be seen from behind. When lifting weights or anything heavy, I use this method of breathing as a bracing method. I teach it to sprinters in the blocks as a bracing system to explode out at the start of the race or when lifting anything. If you are doing an overhead lift, you will need to breathe down and around your core to stabilize. Belly breathing is the most common breath that you will use throughout the day and the primal way to stabilize.

The second breathing sequence to learn is one by the Foundation system. Once you find your proper posture, it teaches you to expand your lungs where your lungs are located. It is not a stress chest breath. This method teaches to expand the breath into your back, widening your lats and wingspan. This system helps with posture. I resonate with this as it is similar to when someone is posturing to fight. They will wing out their lats and make themselves look bigger. I know because I have done it before. Luckily, I am a surfer and my lats are one of my more pronounced muscles. I was playing basketball and had my shirt off, so I was able to avoid the fight.

The third breathing sequence is used to develop energy. It will also get you back into a parasympathetic mode, while developing a greater CO_2 threshold. For this, I use a blend between Pedram Shojai, Brian MacKenzie, Richard LaPlante, and Wim Hof system strategies. Pedram says that all the magic happens on the hold between breaths. So, we pause for 2 seconds between breaths. Wim Hof teaches using more, faster inhales and exhales to warm the body. Brian meshes several techniques and often uses nasal breathing, from the schooling of Free Divers. They do slow, long exhales to increase their CO_2 capacity, allowing them to hold their breath for extended periods. The long, slow exhale is the secret to holding your breath longer. Richard teaches breathing exercises while you are lifting weights to get you even stronger.

Allow me to walk through combining the first sequences.

Do quick nasal inhales and exhales for about 15 seconds. Next, inhale for 5-second durations, pause for 2 seconds, and exhale for 5 seconds. Then repeat. Continue the shorter breaths for the 2 cycles and repeat from the beginning. Build up to doing the entire system 3 times.

Once you have your breath awake and flowing, we can now go into the slow, longer exhale part. Top performers share that creating vivid imagery (visualization) with this breathing pattern will trick the body into creating what you want to happen. So, through breathing and imagery, you can manifest your destiny of the performance you desire.

Troy Casey, the Certified Health Nut, makes it really easy. He just has you breathe in and out with him doing strong breaths. He will take about a dozen or more breaths and have you hold the last breath for about 10 seconds. Just doing focused breathing is the answer to most every health challenge.

One of my former clients was a world record holder in spearfishing and free diving. He taught me years ago that the secret to holding your breath is to exhale very slowly the entire time, so you're not just holding your breath. This is a learned trait. You will learn to get better, or slower and slower, more efficiently letting air out slowly. Concentrating on a long exhale will increase your ability to hold your breath. Find the duration of your exhale by timing yourself to see how slowly you can exhale. Once your find your max, cut it in half using that duration to build up doing the long exhales consecutively. Build it up to 5X. This is some intense stuff and can put some people into what I call la-la land. You may need to pass and take a quick power nap afterward if you overdo it. This breath medicine is a massive lymph flush. So, take heed and train the breath with progression.

I always ask, "Why is it that novice swimmers swim one lap and are completely out of breath?" Most say because they don't know how to swim efficiently, or they are a bit scared. That is part of the answer. When swimming, the water acts as resistance on your exhale. Your lungs actually have to push harder to get rid of the air through blowing bubbles. This is fatiguing to the respiratory system and the main reason you are so out of breath. Swimming and playing a horn instrument are the only two activities that resist the exhale of the breath. These are the best two activities to increase your VO2 max. This is why swimmers have the strongest lungs. A stronger VO2 directly correlates to a healthier body. Breathing into a horn instrument offers this same type of resistance. This is an element of breath strength development that will give you a tremendous advantage and sustained health.

These breathing systems will support you in all performance activities. These systems optimize your alpha levels and get you into more of a high-performance mental flow state, which I will cover in another chapter. These are great ways to stay in the moment, create, and perform.

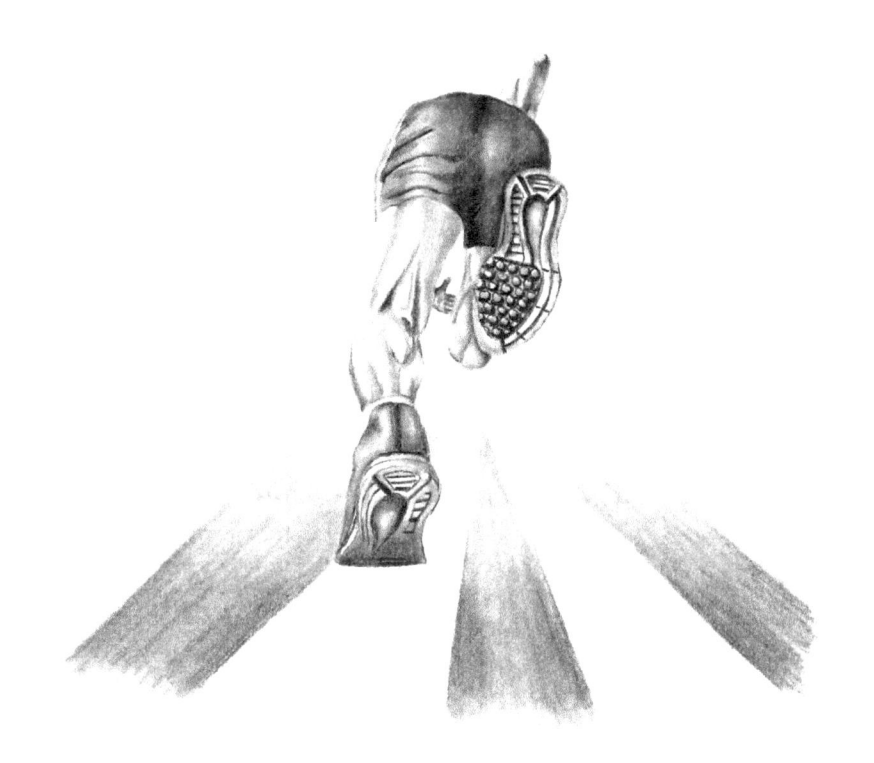

Chapter 5: Speed Techniques.

Learning how to run and move faster is something every athlete trains to do, but we're not taught how to. I played sports my entire life, but until I met Dean Brittenham, I never learned how to run. Thank you again, Dean! Running is something most people don't teach. Most coaches will just say, "Run over here or there," with little or no explanation. When you want to develop more coordination and efficiency, it is important to learn the proper techniques. There is a science behind developing speed, and this section is where you learn specifically how. I write with the same coaching cues, just as though you are doing the drills in front of me.

The maturation of coordination, balance, flexibility, ambidexterity, with quick and powerful turnover, is the focal point of development for speed and a complete elite athlete. Each drill progresses by doing it more efficiently, then faster. We do our movements at a deeper level, focusing on high frequency and high intensity rhythms, mechanics, and posture. Movements are completed through a full range of motion. There are 2 main scientific formulas that validate these teaching techniques to efficiency. The first is:

$$Power = Force \; x \; Distance \; / \; Time$$

The formula for power states, the stronger athlete, with more ROM and the fastest frequency, will have the greatest power output. Think of a rubber band. You pull it back far and it will shoot across the room. Anyone can develop power and speed, faster than ever, through following our program and this equation. Build the fast-twitch Type II muscle fibers with speed and interval development. Just follow the science equations and our speed drills in the next section to get stronger and longer with exceptional results.

$$Velocity = Stride \; length \; x \; Stride \; frequency$$

The same concept applies to velocity. A longer, quicker stride length will generate more velocity. It is pure science. To actually increase your stride length, we run full speed in straight lines. I use some form of a marker to show where you are currently on each stride. You can use a cone, chalk, or tape to measure out 4' to 7' stride lengths, gradually building to a greater range. When you train to increase your stride length, you will get accustomed to running at a greater stride length than normal. This will open your hamstrings and hips up, so when you do your race, you will normalize it to a slightly bigger stride, with a quicker turnover. You will run a faster time according to science. That is why I love science… the formulas don't lie. I set up foam barriers and gradually increase the distance. The foam barriers work well, because if they get stepped on, they give, and you won't hurt your ankles. They also help you develop a more powerful knee drive.

Within the program, there is a progression of exercises from low to high impact. Always start with movements that are lower impact and build to the more explosive ones. Stress the body appropriately to take each athlete out of their coordination comfort zone and continue to allow them to be challenged with new motor movements and ambidexterity. This ensures an athlete will be equally fast and strong moving in any direction during competition. Also, move the body in the various directions by going forward, backward, laterally, horizontally, and vertically with changes of direction. This will prepare the body for any movement necessary during competition.

These warm-ups and workouts are mostly non-linear movements. Skipping, bounding, and shuffling are completed in semicircles or figure 8's. All the ambidexterity exercises allow the athlete to efficiently develop coordination in a circular flow. Athletes need to develop more dimensions for their game. Working out only in straight lines will not get them there. The straight-line development is appropriate during pure sprinting and bursting out of drills.

One of the major differences between ATHLETICISM speed development and other performance programs is the intensity with which each drill is performed. It is all about moving with fast frequency, meaning, to go up and down as fast as possible, with the most efficient technique, both sides equally firing with a full range of motion. A controlled, relaxed coordination, with core and scapular posture awareness, is important. The less time you are on the ground, the faster you will move in every direction. The foot strike paws down so fast, and there is an action with an equal and opposite reaction that occurs, called the stretch shortening cycle. It works just like the rubber band example above. Now the foot strike is not a stomp; it is light and the split second it touches the ground, it is gone. Your arms stay moving as they will facilitate driving the legs.

Another important aspect of our speed and coordination drill is the rhythm. When the athlete skips, there is a beat, the same as in music, called a flamadiddle. Find this rhythm and build the tempo. This rhythm is meant to keep the athlete off the ground, staying fast, light, and nimble. It looks similar to a primal, tribal skipping beat. Learning this rhythm will make some of the best athletes in the world, at first, seem uncoordinated.

Let's simplify the running technique:

1. Running is the foundation for so many of our speed drills. Here are the basics to improve your biomechanics and speed:

    a. Move the opposite arm and leg in synchronicity in a cross-crawl pattern. Your elbows and knees are your motors punching the arms forward and blocking them at about the chin. The big elbows with the hands create an action/reaction, essentially a pulsing action at each end. David Weck would say, "It is a double down, pulsing arm movement, not a swinging arm movement." His WeckMethod Pulsers are a fantastic product to teach you the arm rhythm for running.

    b. The heel comes straight up to the glute, this lifts up the knee while maintaining dorsal flexion in the ankle (toes up). Pretending there is a notch sticking out on the inside of the left knee, the right foot will step over that imaginary notch and paw down explosively to the ground. Dancers are taught to point toes for aesthetics. In order to move more powerfully, athletes drive the knees and have the ankle in dorsal flexion, ready to press down for power and speed. Your knees will not come up past parallel with the ground or too high to slow you down. Running is not a drill, so it is described as a powerful knee drive, not a high knee. Exaggerated movements are done during speed drills and are normalized into efficient movements when looking for top end speed.

c. The foot strike begins with a fast paw down, landing on the front 3/4 of the foot directly under your body. Note, you can and should run heel-toe on a downhill.

d. The heel may touch after the ball of the foot touches and react as a spring as the athlete draws the heel straight up to their glute again. Most of the fastest runners in the world stay on the balls of the feet and the heels do not touch.

e. You want the feet facing forward in the direction you are going. Running with toes pointed outward will slow you down. You may need orthotics if the arches in the feet are collapsing.

f. To begin a sprint on the starting line, you lean forward in a ready position. As you explode out of the blocks and pick up speed, your posture will slowly become more upright in a steady, seamless transition. Once at full speed, any forward lean will initiate at the ankles, not the waist.

2. Proper Posture:
    a. Feet, knees, hips, diaphragm, shoulders are properly lined up, allowing for the head to slightly move right to left toward each foot, with each step.
    b. No counterproductive movement, i.e., no bobble head (rotating right to left), no bending at the waist, over-twisting arms, or twisting hips, no running on the heels or tip of the toes.
    c. The core (center of power) is always moving straight to the finish line. Maintain a strong, relaxed posture with the sternum up, with the forward lean starting at the ankles, not the waist.

3. Arm Action:
    a. The arms are bent at a right angle. Punch forward, pulse, and elbow pulse back behind the body.
    b. The arms stop and block in the front of the body between the chin and the eye level.

c. The thumbs are relaxed upward in front of the body, and they brush back by the hip, with the elbow bent back behind the body.

d. This creates an action, reaction motion for both arms and leg already completed.

4. A strong finish is what every coach looks for, so always run past the finish line. Burst out of every drill into a fast 4- to 6-step sprint. Practicing this now will teach you to finish strong in competition.

Speed & Coordination Drills.

Most just go through the motions and do speed drills about ¼ to ½ speed, in straight lines. The basic speed drills alone are helpful for coordination, but until done properly, you will only get a certain benefit from them. I see so many athletes simply cruise through these movements in warm-ups and workouts. The real benefits come from doing them for speed, with a high intensity, high frequency, through a full range of motion, in the figure 8. When following these drills and cues, your body will become light, coordinated, rhythmic, and explosive, producing the greatest output in your performance. You will get more out of it doing them the ATHLETICISM way.

Below are a series of drills that will give you more bounce and pop in your step. You must train fast to become fast. Below are the fundamental speed drills to facilitate making you faster. You can do all drills forward, sideways (laterally), and backward. You will add change of direction as you progress. Again, burst out of the drills for straight line accelerating and decelerating. These drills will set you up for success and are versatile enough to keep you busy and progressing for decades.

1. High Knee Running With Arms

    This drill is fast running, up and down, slowly moving forward. Heel up, knee up, and toes up. Opposite elbow moves with opposite knee. Have the swing leg heel come all the way up to the glute, driving the knee up and forward, then pawing down on the ball of the foot. Go up and down fast.

2. High Knees Without Arms

    Do just high knees working on the swing leg cycle, relaxing the arms at the side of your body. Stay on the balls of the feet. Doing just arm or leg drills alone, then combining both make the whole stronger.

3. Backward Run

   This is one drill where you must stride out. Heel reaches up to glute and then out behind you. Once comfortable with the movement, start to cover some ground and accelerate backward.

4. Heel Kick-Ups

   a. Maintain your upright posture and do heel kick up to your glutes (butt) to get the knees opened up. Have your knees pointing toward the ground.

   b. Start with only the heels.

   c. Add arms.

5. High Knee Skip

   Bring one bent knee up parallel (halfway) to the ground and the other knee comes all the way up to the chest, shoulder, arm pit area. Maintain proper flamadiddle rhythm, light, nimble, explosive, and not being on the ground long. The best imagery is the way our Native Americans would skip and dance around in a circle, around a campfire with light feet in a celebratory beat. It is a pulsing motion with rhythm. Feel that beat on every leg lift. One knee comes up halfway, the other flexes up all the way, and the feet drive into the ground, getting an instant reaction. Keep your chest up, bringing the knee to the chest, not the chest to the knee.

6. Side Shuffle

    Swing the arms forward and back together while shuffling. To gain momentum, swing both arms up and back, coordinating with the shuffle of the legs. Use the same blocking on the forward and backward swing, as these are your momentum makers to get you more speed. Keep the center of gravity low, through the entire duration. Stay on the balls of your feet. Keep the feet quiet, not clicking them together. Allow each foot to generate its own speed.

7. Side Shuffle With Change of Direction

    When shuffling up about 5 steps and back 2, anticipate the change of direction by leaning back in the direction you will change toward. This will keep you balanced and facilitate in a quicker change of direction. The moment you change directions, make sure the hands are back behind the body so they can pulse and drive them forward with the hips to accelerate you in the new direction. Also, just prior to changing directions, plant the feet and explode out, with no extra steps.

8. Parallel Bounding

    This is one of my favorite drills because it offers everything for everyone. An easy way to describe it is to straddle a line and keep each foot on the same side of the line. It is similar to wide running, where you bound, with each foot landing on the same side of the line they started. Stay on the balls of the feet and explode or bound from one leg to the next. Keep the leg tucked and drive the knee up and out. Go for height first and progress with width, landing softly, seamlessly transitioning to the next leg. Maintain posture, core strength, and the arm action of opposite arm to opposite leg, to drive the legs. Any weak links in your foot or leg will show by your leg giving out a bit, not allowing you to bound explosively. Maintain balance and develop explosive strength on each leg individually. Bounding is one of the best exercises any athlete can do to develop power in each leg individually.

9. Ankle Hops

    This drill is similar to a jumping rope motion. Starting with both legs, simply hopping up and down from the ankles only. Develop the strength in the plantar flexion of the ankle. Be light and quick with each hop, keeping the upper body and hips relatively still. Start with no arms, then add arms for more bounce in the hop. The arms would swing in front of you and slightly upward, blocking in the air and resetting to hop again.

10. Fast Feet

    Keep the head, chest, and hands up in ready position and drop the hips down. You see this a lot used as a fast feet football drill. From the balls of your feet, move the feet as fast as possible up and down, with the fastest smallest steps possible. This is over-speed development for the nervous system. The faster they fire, the more fast-twitch fibers will be developed. You should be able to hear the speed of the feet moving them forward, in and out.

11. Skipping for Height

    Skip then transition into a heel/toe jump for height. Use the arms, hips, and ankles and accelerate into the heel/toe action to get an explosive reaction of a jump for height off one leg. It is a quick down/up action to accelerate through the ankle and foot. Skip as high as you can, absorb the landing, skipping and accelerating into the next jump on the same leg. Then skip and jump off the other leg.

12. Skipping for Distance

    Use the same skip, then transition into a heel/toe jump for distance. Use the arms, hips, and ankles and accelerate into the heel/toe action to get an explosive reaction of a jump, but now for distance, not height. Alternate legs. This is a more advanced speed drill to develop power, so do it toward the end of the list, making sure you are warm and can maximize it. Skipping is such a fundamental exercise and it is amazing to progress with it. It will bring out power in your legs.

13. Karaoke

    These are essentially lateral, crossover steps in front of the body, then behind the body. Moving laterally to your right, side-step the right leg out, the other back crossing it behind the right leg, then step out with the right leg and cross the left in front of the right leg. Continue this lateral movement with a rhythm. Separate the hips from the shoulders by putting your arms straight out, with making a straight line with the arms in the direction you are moving. So, the hips and feet move fast, and the upper body stays still. Start the drill slow and increase foot and hip speed by the end.

14. Side Shuffle for Height

    a. Pulse the arms forward and back with the legs as they shuffle together and apart. On the forward arm movement, block them at the chin level and jump or shuffle up and over, through the block as high and far as possible.

    b. Want to get sport specific? This is a perfect volleyball blocking drill. Just extend the arms up to mimic a block. The feet should shuffle jump from right where they landed, not allowing for any extra steps that would delay the jump.

15. Serpentine

    This is a fast foot drill for accuracy. You serpentine in and around the barriers. First, you face forward moving right to left. Next, you would face the middle moving through the course forward and back. Last, you would face backward. This would get you moving backward, right to left using your peripheral vision.

16. Heel Kick-Ups, High Knee, Stride and Sprint

    This is where we seamlessly put it all together. Do Heel Kick-Ups With Arms and transition into High Knees With Arms, exaggerated stride it out, then condense it into a sprint. Condense the exaggerated movements into a more efficient sprint and for about 30 yards. Your stride should be longer and faster. The Heel Kicks and High Knees will be done along the semicircle of the outside of the barriers. The Stride and Sprint are in a straight line.

ATHLETICISM

Chapter 6: Power.

Power Running: Let's convert that newfound speed into power. Once the foundation is developed and the athlete is stable, long, completely warmed up with Speed Drills, they can progress to power running and jumping. This power brings another dimension to your workouts and game. Plus, it is another fun part of our program. The power running comes with the knee drives, ideally over barriers. I use foam barriers to force the athlete to drive with their knees. You can also roll up a towel to use as a barrier if you don't have the proper equipment. As your level advances, we will do resistance speed drills and running with the stretching belts around your waist or pelvis.

We have 6-, 9-, and 14-inch heights, that can be used inside or outside. The barriers are set 3 to 4 feet apart for the drills. We set up 9 to12 of them on each semicircle. These barriers teach you to use your cognitive skills as well. You learn to count the number of barriers, changing direction on the right number. This teaches you to anticipate and stay in the moment.

The different size barriers teach you to have awareness in driving the knees when running and using the arms and elbows to further propel yourself to get over each barrier. The barriers just get you to pick up your feet and force you to do a proper swing leg cycle, while moving in all directions.

A more powerful and efficient knee drive equates to faster running.

Let's start by setting up the course in our semicircles ( ). Again, you are going up and down more than moving fast forward. If you ran fast forward, you would outrun the course, knocking over the barriers. The focus is to keep your composure and stay in the course, developing the coordination in your legs to be powerful and accurate. Be creative in the way you work out and develop the whole body. You can expand the course as your power level increases.

Here are your Power Running Drills.

1. One Step
    a. Run through the barriers straight ahead with 1 step between each barrier. Alternate the first step, starting with the right, then left.
2. Two Steps
    a. Run through the barriers with 2 steps in between each barrier. Alternate your lead leg. Keep the arms moving to help keep the legs in rhythm.
3. Two Steps, Side Steps
    a. Two steps, side steps laterally. Face the middle on each side, and you will work both sides equally.

b. Do not do crossover steps on this drill. Step next to your other foot.

4. One-Step Crossovers

   a. The first step is a powerful crossover step over the first barrier, driving the knee down the line.

   b. Do 1 step in between each barrier, so the second step is a side step.

   c. Add a change of direction for a more advanced drill. Go up 6, back 2 with crossovers on each step where your change direction.

Start with these running drills and see your body develop more coordination, rhythm, and power. Make sure to sprint out of the last barrier to learn acceleration and to finish strong. Again, coaches love to see strong finishes to drills. That strong finish will carry over into your finishing strong during competition. The next progression to power running is doing this same routine on an incline.

When doing stride length work, set up the barriers progressively 6 to 9 feet apart in a straight line. The last several barriers take the stride way out of your comfort zone. When you go back to your normal stride, the stride length will be slightly longer with the same fast turnover. This will make you run faster.

Power Jumping: There are endless drills to do over the barriers. Make sure to follow proper squatting, posture, and tracking of the knees, into a condensed range, with an explosive jump movement. When jumping, make sure to channel the energy up in the direction you want to go. It is really about converting the strength developed and directing it upward to defy gravity. As I previously mentioned, the power movements in semicircles release endorphins and develop the Whole Body Whole Brain plasticity. This connects the athlete to a deeper flow state.

There are several different types of jumps to teach. They include: deep knee bend jumps, quarter knee bend jumps, ankle hops, change of direction jumps, jumps in every direction, and one leg hops. On all jumps, the athlete must maintain the proper technique, posture, and tracking. Newton's third law is, "For every action, there is an equal and opposite reaction." Again, we're following science. When you are set to jump and do a vertical leap test, drop and load down quick, to go up quickly, using the arms explosively for best results. This develops that quick eccentric, change of energy and direction, stretch shortening for optimal power.

The little corrections make all the difference on the power output. Most individuals do a little jump to prepare themselves to do a bigger one. I call it jumping before you jump. We want to get rid of that first little jump to develop more eccentric strength. So, you want to learn to prepare for the next consecutive jump when you are in the air. Any extra jump or step, regardless of how small, will slow you down in a game.

This eccentric power is needed for jumping and all explosive moves. The concept is to load the muscles so the stretch-shortening cycle takes place precisely when you want it. The cues I use are to be light and nimble, absorbing and re-firing quickly with no extra steps. The athlete must jump with integration of their arms, hips, and ankles. The arms will be in a quick power, pulsing, uppercut and block about the chin level. When in midair, make sure to bring the arms back down toward your side, so you are ready to drive and pulse them up again on the next jump. As your energy keeps moving up to the peak of the jump, the arms will block at your chin and circle out and back down, so you are coiled to jump quickly again once you land.

Maintaining the proper posture will help avoid bending at the waist, using your back as the major jump muscle group. So many athletes lack the flexibility and posture to get into the proper position and injure their spine in the process. This is why we do so much work on proper squatting, posture, core, and flexibility. Proper position, driving from the stable core and foundation, will bring you a more powerful jump.

The stronger athlete with…

1. no weak links
2. proper flexibility
3. the most fast-twitch muscle fibers
4. the quickest, most efficient turnover

…will be the most powerful athlete. We must combine the entire equation and more when developing the Whole Body.

Maintain proper posture so you can see what is going on around you, where to make the play, pass, and so on. The spatial awareness, thinking skills, vision, and peripheral vision are all developed when jumping with the barriers. I will hold my hands up flashing various numbers of fingers in the air. You will call out how many fingers I'm holding up while doing the barriers. This is one way to get you to look up at the field of play, not down at your feet. It is another form of Neuro Stacking as you must stay on course, keep your head up, and call out certain numbers. When you miss a barrier, it is considered an unforced error, turnover, essentially, a point for the opponents. After a few push-ups, you will not want to make another mistake of knocking over another barrier. This brain plasticity comes alive with the body movements and you get more efficient. Now we can finally see all the pieces of the puzzle coming together.

Power Jumps include:

1. Double Leg Hops Straight Ahead
    a. Use your arms, hips, and ankles.
    b. Land on and jump off both feet at the same time.
    c. Be light, nimble, and explosive.
    d. Do a longer jump at the end of the course, jumping over the last 2 barriers.
2. Lateral Double Leg Hops
    a. Lean in the direction you are jumping.
    b. Jump off both feet at the same time.
    c. Do a big jump over the last 2 barriers.
3. Lateral Double Leg Hops With Change of Direction
    a. Go up 6 barriers and back 2.
    b. No double jumps or shifting your feet before you change direction. Just land and jump out of it. Time your arms, hips, ankles, and lean in the direction you are going or wanting to go. When preparing for any change of direction, anticipate the lean and jump back the other direction.
4. Single Leg Hops Forward
    a. Track the second toe and knee
    b. Use your hips and arms to propel the body
5. Single Leg Hops Lateral
    a. Use your hips and arms to propel the body and lean in the direction you are going.

6. Single Leg Hops Laterally With Change of Direction
    a. Use your hips and arms to propel the body and anticipate the change of direction by leaning that way.

    Once you go through all the speed and power drills, the more advanced athletes will finish with big jumps over a waist-high, 48" foam barrier. We do forward, lateral, and backward jumps over the barriers. I set up the course with 3 barriers.

7. Forward Jumps.
    a. Use your arms, hips, and ankles to jump.
    b. Bend knees and lightly absorb the landing and re-fire.
    c. Make sure the knees track over the second toe, and don't waiver or collapse inward.
    d. Go down 3. Stop, rest, turn around, and come back.
    e. Rest and repeat.
    f. This time rotate 180° on the third barrier, land, and come back to where you started.
    g. Next, on the third barrier, in the air, rotate 180° the other direction, land, and with no extra steps, jump back to where you started. Practice turning right and left on the change of direction.

8. Lateral Jumps

a. Lean in the direction you are jumping

b. Jump over the 3 barriers, rest, and return facing the same direction

c. Next, on the third jump, land and return to where you started without any extra jumps or steps.

d. I call this back over the middle. You change direction on the middle barrier and the third barrier. You start and finish at the same spot. Do not use any extra steps in any of the jumps. Anticipate all change of directions.

Are some of you reading this and thinking, how is jumping over and back so monumental? Or, how are these speed drills so much better from other track programs. First, I challenge you to do the program. It sounds way easier than it actually is to do. There are incredible hormonal releases, nerve and muscle responses with our program. Everything is thought through, and here is a list to confirm it all.

1. Foam barriers are soft so you won't get hurt if you step on them
2. Non-linear
3. Course is set up in a figure 8
4. Progression
5. Massive menu
6. Exact biomechanical cues on every step

7. Up and down fast or not on the ground for long
8. You can run a big group at the same time
9. You can have different levels and ages in the same group
10. You must think and count while doing the drills
11. You sprint out of the drills
12. It is the athlete versus their own coordination

I could keep going, but I think you get the point. Everything is just done right.

Next are the more advanced jumps. You can do a 3- or 5-barrier course with this same jump course. Spread the barriers apart to increase difficulty. Add a hill for another degree of difficulty. These barrier jump drills are where we see the body become light, nimble, and explosive.

In addition to our barriers, we recently rolled out a new jump rope that is done with three people. The ATHLETICISM American Jump Band is so fun and versatile for developing coordination and eccentric power. You will want to experience it.

1. Straddle – Side – Straddle – Side. Start on a straight line. Straddle the line. Hop both feet over to the right side of the line. Hop back to straddle the line. Then hop both feet over to the left side of the line. Repeat. Continue to speed up the feet moving

forward, then backward, up, and down the line. This can be quite challenging to keep in a fast rhythm.

2. On the straight line, move laterally, doing fast feet drills up, with your feet moving over the line and back. Make sure the feet are moving back and forth at the same time. Next alternate feet on either side of the line. Move the feet back and forth, as fast as possible. Even though the feet are moving fast, forward and back, they are not moving fast laterally.

3. For these exercises, use chalk or find 2 lines that cross in a + shape. Put one foot in each opposite quadrant. Make sure to alternate the first turn from right, then to left. Do 10 turns one direction (right), rest, then do 10 turns the other direction (left).

    a. ¼ Turns with whole body
    b. ¼ Turns with lower half of your body
    c. ½ Turns with whole body
    d. ½ Turns with lower half of your body
    e. Make sure to have your arms out like an airplane to open your chest to the direction you will turn. This will allow your lower body to do ½ turns.
    f. Full Body 360° Turn to Right
    g. Full Body 360° Turn to Left
        i. Keep your head over your feet during the rotation. Land with the feet as close to the

same spot and direction they faced at the start of the jump.

Learning rotational balance and power through the core is a major part of sports. When you can learn to isolate the hips and shoulder and connect that coil or torque via the figure 8, you will be the most accurate and powerful hitter, thrower, or server. The full 360° rotational moves used to be done only by basketball players or NFL running backs. Now you see surfing, snowboarding, skiing, and many more sports all doing aerial 360° plus moves. This is the coordination and ambidexterity development we are looking for in the body. Make sure to train with progression and mix up your workouts.

This run and jump program is fantastic and will get you faster and more powerful than ever. This course never gets old and will keep challenging you at every level.

Make sure to add in your toe raises to strengthen your tibialis anterior muscle. This is a big area of focus for power and jumping athletes to get that action and reaction. I love to use the Aaron Mattes Ankle Exerciser. You need the joint stability products before you go into the prime mover exercises of squats.

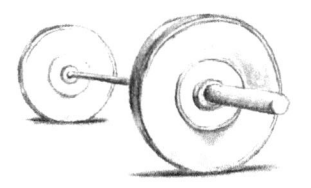

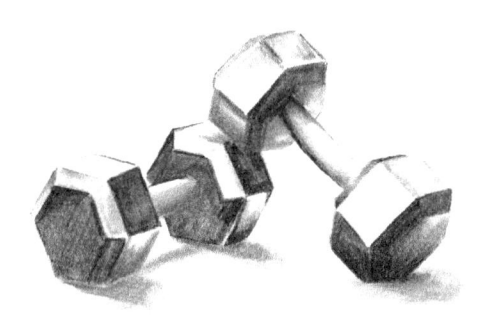

Chapter 7: Olympic Lifting for Sports & Squats.

In Europe, many consider Olympic lifting the most athletic sport in the world. This is because the strength and power output of an athlete can be quantifiably measured pound for pound. The major lifts are the clean and jerk, and the snatch and squat. In the 2008 Beijing Olympics, the 94 KG lifters clean and jerked 227 KG. That means they lifted it up to their chest into a squat, stood, then lifted it over their head. The conversion from kilos to pounds is 2.2. This equates to 227 x 2.2 = 499.4 lbs. This is the power potential of the human body when properly trained, and it is only getting stronger. If you watched or listened to any of our Go Beyond Summit on Human Performance, my O-lifting coach, Jerzy Gregorek talks about all the benefits.

Jerzy taught me all about developing a foundational strength base and strength in the pelvic floor through deep squats. There are fundamental lifts that everyone should be able to do. You see it in kids at an early age. They are the best at squatting. Somehow, we often lose that movement. Squatting is the base of everything. It gets you top to bottom strength. It is ambidexterity to the fullest. Each side of your body has to be as balanced as possible. First use your body weight when squatting, cleaning, and jerking. For more advanced athletes, build up to lifting approximately your body weight or more.

If you recognize Jerzy's name, you may be a Tim Ferris fan, reader, or watch TED Talks. On the main stage at TED, Tim Ferris gave his talk and cited Jerzy as one of the top 10 most successful people he has ever met in his life. That is quite an accolade from such a well-traveled and extensive researcher as Tim Ferris. I saw Jerzy's talents years ago when I paid him to train me out of Gold's Gym in Venice Beach, California. I had been in the business enough years to know who had the "it factor." One of the major lessons I learned watching him work was understanding how medicinal it is to rehab all clients through these lifts. I had just torn my ACL and was rehabbing it after surgery. A football player had a dislocated shoulder and Jerzy brought him back stronger than ever. One of the smallest guys had been O lifting since he was 9 and could outlift all of us, effortlessly. Jerzy could pick apart every weakness and give an O lifting exercise to correct it.

The philosophy of Europeans is more about proper strength development, prior to playing a sport. They have certain strength benchmarks that they meet to prevent injuries and improve performance. We need to adopt a balance of this philosophy. Our culture typically just goes out and plays sports for hours without ever lifting, stretching, or preparing for the activity.

I understand that many people reading this book are not into doing heavy Olympic lifts (O lifts). What I do know is that we can learn a lot from this system of lifting. We can also get tremendous results duplicating many of the full range of motion lifts and their movement systems, without needing heavy weights. I can walk into any gym and see people doing half squats. The knees come alive when you drop all the way down into a full squat. Just the concept of working towards a full range of motion should be enough to get you to understand. You don't just do biceps curls at a right angle. O lifters are the strongest athletes in the world. They lift more weight daily then anyone, and they do full squats.

You can use a stretching belt, towel, or dowel rod for learning how to do an overhead squat. For all of us, it is more about developing posture and a full range of motion. O lifting for sport establishes a foundation with integrity of tracking the knees properly. O lifts are best used for balancing and stabilizing an individual. Overhead squats are the ideal support lifts to reshape the posture of the spine, to create a top-to-bottom stable athlete. This strength development with your arms overhead makes you more flexible and stronger. Plus, it provides tremendous overhead stability for all hitting and throwing sports, like tennis, baseball, volleyball, and so on.

There is a balance you must find when developing athletes. ATHLETICISM will provide an actual program so the athlete won't have to spend 5 hours on their sport every day. Now, they can schedule their day without worrying about overtraining. Instead of a professional athlete playing one sport all day, they can follow our ATHLETICISM programs to make significant gains.

I am an O lifting coach for sport, not for competition. The movements taught are the major support lifts. We are not even coming close to the heavy weights needed to compete in the competition. I do highly recommend getting custom orthotics during the developmental stages, before competing, and for general overall health and injury prevention. "An ounce of prevention is worth a pound of cure,"[16] says Tom Brady.

---

[16] Brady T. *The TB12 Method*. New York, NY: Simon & Schuster; 2017.

Steven Dreyer, DC, from Newport Spine & Sport, makes my orthotics, and they have saved my feet, knees, and back as I have gotten older. O lifters use stiff, raised heel shoes that offer lots of support, but there is nothing better than having custom orthotics made. I use my orthotics in every activity I do.

Here is a more detailed checklist of squat cues, expanding on earlier cues:

1. Breathe down to the lowest part of your abdominals while drawing the breath around your low back to support the entire hips and spine. This broadening of the core will support compression around you from the hips to the diaphragm. So many people get back injuries from not breathing and supporting their core properly.

2. When doing squats or O lifts, hold the breath through much of the lift, maintaining this abdominal pressure. Breathe in before the squat or movement. On the way out of the lift, slowly let air out on the way up, exhaling it all out when completed.

3. To access Qi energy at the center-of-power of your body, maintain the intent of deep, belly breathing to release and draw in energy to and from the core.

4. Breathe down to the lowest part of your abdominals while drawing the breath around your low back to support the entire hips and spine.

When doing squats, go through the checkpoints below first. Once you have a grasp of these, your setup will be instantaneous:

1. Find perfect posture and line up your feet in a straight line.
2. Place legs hip-to-shoulder width apart. Add about a 1" lift underneath your heels, if needed, for beginners. This lift will allow a more stable, upright squat, so you don't rock backward.
3. Breathe down and around for abdominal support (hold breath through the squat and exhale toward the top). Repeat.
4. When squatting with just your body weight, cross arms up and out in front of you, to keep the thoracic spine and sternum upright.
5. Keep your head looking straight throughout the entire movement.
6. Stay equal on each side. If one foot is in front of the other, or if the bar overhead is rotating to one side, you need to correct it. Have someone make sure you stay lined up on the lower and upper body.
7. Bend your knees and sit all the way down onto your heels. You want a full range of motion (ROM). If your weight is too far forward or backward, the body will fall that direction when loaded. Plus, if forward, there will be added pressure on the knees that you want to

avoid during strength development. Use the 3-point contact triangle to balance weight distribution through your heel, ball of foot, and the little toe side of the ball of the foot.

8. Track kneecap over second toe through the entire motion and keep your arches strong with three touch points of the foot connecting. The touch points are your heel and the inside and outside ball of the foot.

9. Stand up as you are, pushing and driving through the eye of the heels.

10. Do not hyper extend knees at top. Just lock them out to the straight position.

11. Maintain safety. The lifter has the right of way, so stay off the platform and clear of their area. Most gyms have the entire floor padded, so wherever there is a rack or bar, someone can be lifting. You must be spatially aware. Spotters communicate where and when they will support the lifter prior to the lift. When doing overhead lifts, the lifter can drop the bar in front or behind them for their safety.

Any collapsing of the hips, knees, or wavering of the knees is a sign of a weak link in the knees, core, hips, legs, or feet, so maintain control and composure. The main support lifts used are front squats, overhead squats, and overhead press. We do not initially do back squats, since many athletes do not have the strength or flexibility to load the weight at that angle. Proper front and overhead squats and building a more stable foundation will save many back injuries. You can add back squats as strength progresses.

To build a foundation, build up to 10 sets of 10 repetitions of front squats and 10 sets of 10 overhead squats. Gravity will provide enough resistance initially, then slowly add weight. Lunges and step-ups are also part of building a strength foundation. Remember muscle endurance and resiliency are part of the foundation strength phase.

Once the foundation is built, Dr. Michael Yessis will say to do 1 X 20 Repetition Max (RM) in all lifts and jumps. This will allow you to have a "specialized strength"[17] level to improve your performance. I interviewed him in 2015 for our Go Beyond Summit, and he shared this breakthrough. Combining the foundation with 1 X 20 RM is amazing for elevating performance.

---

[17] Yesses M. *The Revolutionary 1 X 20 RM Strength Training Program*. California, USA: Sports Training, Inc; 2014.

Chapter 8: Stretching.

Just as Dean was a pioneer in performance, so is Aaron Mattes in stretching. He created one of the most effective assisted and unassisted stretching methods available. I was fortunate that Dean already knew Aaron and was working with and doing athletic development with Aaron's son for professional sports. My first day working with Dean we did AIS stretches. I have seen so many injuries over the past 22 plus years from lack of flexibility. Many of them come in after yoga or Crossfit because they didn't have a foundation and pushed themselves too hard. To combat this, the Aaron Mattes Active Isolated Stretching (AIS) is our preferred stretching method bringing pliability and stability. It is a system that can warm you up for yoga or any activity. It will improve your performance and facilitate in a speedy recovery.

AIS has been deemed the fountain of youth by many of my clients. I start with assessing the athlete on their ROM in multiple movements and stretches. With the assessment, I have information as to where to correct and treat. "I began to dissect movement and gather strength exercise protocols designed to specifically strengthen muscles that surround regions that span and support joints,"[18] by Aaron Mattes. Aaron developed one of the most incredibly effective stretching and joint strengthening systems. The AI stretching principals are based on reciprocal innervation. The agonist

---

[18] Mattes AL. Active Isolated Strengthening: The Mattes Method. Aaron Mattes Therapy; 2006.

is contracted while the antagonist is inhibited and relaxed, so it can be stretched. This muscle counterbalance is exactly how the body functions during motion, so this system makes the most sense to us. The body responds with incredible flexibility of the muscle and joint.

Aaron Mattes believes the muscles have a 2-second breath. Just hold the stretch for 2 seconds, then release and do it again. To optimize the stretch, repeat about 10 times on each angle, for each muscle. Less repetition and a shorter hold are needed before competition, making it a fantastic warm-up. Breathing is an important part of stretching. Exhale on the stretch. This method pumps blood, oxygen, and nutrients to the body and fascia. This stretch on specific muscles is also a major lymph flush. This system is so effective, and it allows you to exactly pinpoint where the tight areas are located. It opens the medial, lateral, and belly of the muscle covering all 3 angles of every muscle. The repetition of each stretch will gain range of motion instantly.

This system is an active stretch and can be used as a warm-up, recovery, or simply to gain range of motion. There are also instant medicinal benefits, including flushing the lymph, ridding pain and soreness, and more. A diversion of circulation is a major part of why people have pain. AIS will increase blood flow and get the energy flowing back on track. Bones follow muscles, so this system will be an integral part of improving posture. Remember, this is an active stretch so you must actively lift your leg, then assist with the hands or belt when used. Each stretch also talks to your nervous system and brain, preparing you for sport. Static stretching is known to diminish performance prior to sport, but AIS will improve it.

When doing the unassisted stretches, it is important to have a stretching belt or towel to assist with the lower body stretches. Make sure to stretch all 3 angles of medial, lateral, and belly of the muscle. To do this you can have the belt straight or wrap around the inside or outside of the leg to assist in rotation so proper angles are stretched. Once you are thoroughly stretched, we will cover joint stability, as every great stretching program needs stability exercises and development to support the stretch.

There is a misconception in yoga classes. Yoga is an art, and you need to prepare for class, the same as you would for sport. Just because you are amazing at stretching and breathing in a yoga class, does not mean you can skip a pre-stretch to prepare for class. This proper warm-up will allow you a more productive yoga class.

In my clinic, I do nerve stability first, then AI stretching. The combinations are remarkably effective. You feel like you are floating after a treatment. Posture is restored and injuries disappear. Since I do not adjust clients, I use distraction techniques, using gravity is another great way to stretch. Hanging from a bar will also help align and decompress the spine and hips. The results are unbelievable. You, too, can achieve these amazing results with the AI stretching unassisted version, where you stretch on your own and use a belt. I always assess, correcting through stability and stretching, prior to any speed or power movements.

I recommend going to StretchingUSA.com to purchase any of their books to learn more about this incredible stretching and joint stability system. Kelly Carter, DAOM, has built his entire practice around this AIS system with celebrities like Adam Carolla. This system gets impressive results.

Chapter 9: Balance Development.

Balance is one of the most overlooked components of athletic development. If you don't have balance, you can't do anything effectively. I want all my clients to develop superior balance. It is one of the easiest systems to train. Start by balancing on each leg individually. You can easily do ambidexterity development, joint stability work, and balance work from the ground. Standing on an unstable surface will garner better balance for you. It wakes up the nervous system and develops the stabilizers or smaller muscles that support the joints. The joints will get stronger due to all the smaller muscle groups working to support the joints. Everyone works the big prime movers, but most people's weak links are their joints. So, stabilize the weak links and the whole body becomes stronger.

This is my secret weapon for being stronger than guys twice my size on the basketball court. I am quick and nimble, but my balance and lateral stability are far superior to theirs. I can easily lean in for position and move them out of the way. If they throw a hip at me, I can out stabilize them laterally, or I can avoid the hit and keep their momentum going in that direction while I get into position. It takes stability, balance, and timing to exploit an athlete's weakness.

Here are my go-to balance products:

1. BOSU ball
2. Gym ball

3. Dyna-Disc
4. Foam pillow
5. Board rock
6. Extreme balance board
7. Figure 8 Board (rotational balance)
8. Waff

Start your foundational balance exercises by balancing on a painted line on the ground. While standing on both legs, look every direction (right, left, up, down, and close your eyes for 10 seconds). Your brain will soon learn better proprioception and adapt with proper progression. Next, balance on only one leg and challenge the proprioception by looking all directions. Then do the above program on a BOSU ball.

I'll start with the BOSU ball as it has revolutionized the health, fitness, and performance industries. David Weck, the founder of the BOSU ball, has invented about a dozen incredible products. The BOSU ball is a standout favorite for developing balance and stability equally on both sides of the body. You can train the upper and lower body. Most every major gym has a BOSU ball in it. And if they don't, they need to get it. David brought one of the first BOSU balls ever made to Scripps Clinic in the late 1990s. Dean actually validated it and showed him a bunch of exercises to do on it. David is another forward thinker who is completely ambidextrous. He masters his products and sells millions of them.

Having superior balance will allow a higher level of performance. When balanced, an individual will typically perform with a higher percentage of accuracy. Stabilizing the joints through endurance development, balancing for long durations on the ball, will also be helpful for injury prevention. Simply balancing is developing the proprioceptive sense through position and movement. You want to teach your body to learn where it is in space.

As high-level performers, we want to heighten all our senses and not just rely on one. We have proprioceptors on our skin and throughout our entire body, vision, and inner ear. Centering yourself is one of the most important aspects of performance development. When you take away the vision, the other senses get stronger, making the whole body stronger.

Danny Putnam was a supplemental first-round MLB draft pick out of Stanford University. He was the only player in the dorms at that time who had a BOSU ball in his dorm room. He would blindfold himself and do all the above balance exercises every day. With his ATHLETICISM Whole Body Whole Brain development, he made it to "the bigs."

There are virtually endless ambidexterity exercises you can do on a BOSU ball. At a minimum, get or use a BOSU ball and a gym ball. There are endless exercises to maximize your investment and performance.

The Figure 8 Board is the best tool for teaching spinning and landing in each direction. Make sure to spin on each leg in each direction. Just stand and move your hips in a figure 8. Your energy will shift instantly. When you do it on one side, do the same on the other. I have used this product for years. It is on my favorites list without a doubt. This simple movement is the key to every hitting or throwing sport. It is the key to martial arts, surfing, and most activities. When you flow in a figure 8, the body responds so well.

One of the founders, Jack Broudy, is a professional tennis instructor. He is one of the first coaches I wanted my daughter to take lessons from. He taught her to hit from her body, not her arms, using her core with a figure 8. He has produced many of the top junior players over the past several decades. You can learn his system at BroudyTennis.com. This movement system is not just for tennis players. It is applicable to all hitting and throwing sports. Learning to move the body in a figure 8 is one of the most important components to performance. The second I go to throw or hit a ball, I derive all my power from the core, use the coil, and torque to get the most power from this figure 8 movement.

We can do a workout in a figure 8, juggling and creating a figure 8, or hitting and going through using the figure 8. I can't emphasize enough how big the figure 8 is in every aspect of biomechanics, movement, and performance. When you have superior balance in the figure 8, everything gets better.

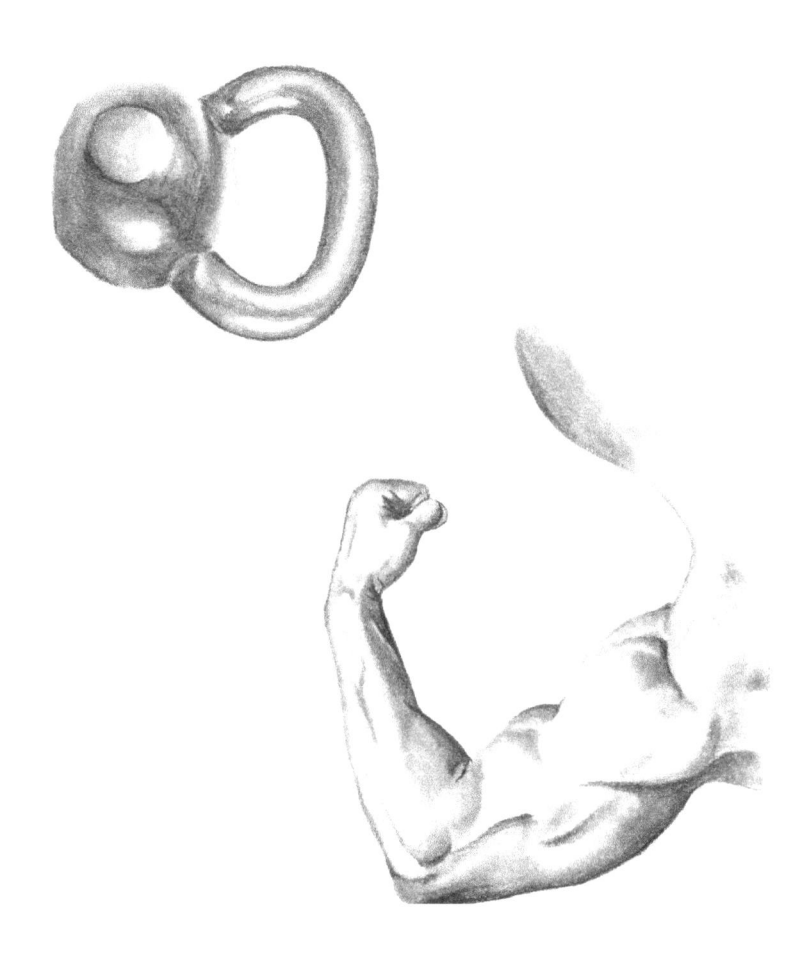

Chapter 10: Kettlebells.

Kettlebells for breakfast?! Well, I don't eat them, but I do use them daily. One of my colleagues, Steve Cotter, is considered one of the first guys to bring the kettlebell (KB) into the US. He mastered KBs and introduced them to me over 15 years ago, and now they are sold at Target. I took the initial course he taught and did numerous private sessions with him. I love working with KBs as they connect my core, and they are a feel good, Whole Body movement system.

There is an acceleration and deceleration component with the weight that gets you unbelievably strong. I can flow and get in a great rhythm swinging them. They have all different weights, so beginners can be safely introduced to them. My working weight for two- and one-arm swings is 72 lbs. It keeps me on my game. When strengthening with KBs, there are also several eye-hand exercises you can do that other systems don't allow. The unilateral overhead stability and endurance is unmatched.

The proper body position to swing KBs is similar to squatting. Maintain the same proper cues (feet in line, posture, etc.) that we learned in squatting, to set yourself up to lift any type of weight. The KBs are a dynamic tool to develop strength. Developing unilaterally and bilaterally (with a kettlebell in each hand) allows the athlete to work both sides at a deeper level. This will definitely get the heart rate up as we increase volume and weight. Start with a smaller, lightweight KB and follow the proper techniques and movement system first.

Safety is the utmost importance when swinging KBs. Make sure the individual has a defined area where others stay clear and don't go in front of the lifter. Even the pros have accidents, so clear an area. Have a heightened awareness of picking the KB up between the legs and setting it back down between the legs. No getting casual and swinging it to the side of the leg. If the KB hits the knee, it can be very painful and cause a big contusion or a more serious injury. Also, cue the athlete not to let go of the KB when doing a swing or snatch lift. Even though the grip is light, the index finger and thumb should hook the KB. Don't release until the KB is back safely on the ground.

Kettlebells are a dynamic way to gain strength in the core and posterior chain. The hips hinge and thrust so the core does all the work. The arms are just an extension of the body. Hold the kettlebell with a grip just firm enough not to let go, hooking the index finger and thumb in the corner of the KB, as your locking mechanism. If your grip is squeezed too tightly, you will fatigue rapidly. This goes the same for the rest of the body. Stabilize the core by breathing down and around the lumbo-pelvic area, and don't expend too much energy on other areas involved. When doing one arm lifts, hold the KB at the opposite corner. Follow the KB all the way through the lift with the opposite arm, making sure the KB is fluid and not jerking at any point during the swing. Once you become highly efficient with this movement system, add an appropriate and gradual increase in weight. KBs already have big jumps in weight so start off slow and build a foundation with volume. Use this more as a coordinated movement system that will develop more endurance strength in an athletic position and mental toughness. We are not looking to be a competition lifter, but we do want to strengthen the entire body with all the various lifts that can be done with a KB. Here are several lifts to get you started.

1. KB Warm-Up

a. Pass the KB in figure 8's between and around the legs. Maintain proper posture with a horse stance (feet wide apart and knees bent). There are unlimited lifts you can graduate to doing.

2. KB Two-Arm Swing

    a. Grip the handle of the KB, hooking the index and thumb. Maintain proper posture, lift, and drive the power through the heels.

    b. Swing can go as high as directly over your head. Start by swinging it up to your stomach, then your chest, and progress accordingly.

    c. These are designed to be endurance exercises, so you can build up to going until you need to stop.

3. KB One-Arm Swing

    a. Grip the handle at the corner and swing.

    b. The opposite hand follows, maintaining a fluid flow up and back.

4. One-Arm Clean

    a. Make it a seamless flip of the KB to the back side of your arm.

5. The catch or top part of the movement keeps the arm close to the body with the thumb almost toward the center of the chest.

6. One-Arm Press

    a. Start from the top of the clean, or racked, position (held at chest/shoulder) and press upward.

    b. Lock the arm out, above your head.

    c. Use the core and legs to help with the press.

7. One-Arm Snatch

    a. From a swing, make it a seamless flip of the KB to the back side of your arm.

    b. Your arm will lock out above your head.

    c. On the down swing, absorb it with your core, hips, and power muscles.

8. Upright Row

    a. Balance on one leg, hinge forward at the waist, and lift the KB with the opposite arm, rowing it up toward the side of your stomach. Switch arms after each set of 20.

The benefits of kettlebells are unlimited. As you get stronger, you can progress to a KB in each hand, swinging them at the same time. It is an athletic, coordinated full body movement system supporting the lumbo-pelvic area. The results are developed quickly without spending a lot of time lifting. Just a 10-minute workout can garner tremendous results.

There is a ton of material in this Whole Body section. It could not be more teed up for you to use this program to go beyond. Let's start learning the Whole Brain programs.

Part III. Whole Brain Coordination.

Chapter 11: Whole Brain Exercises.

Now that you know the proper nutrition, awareness, and coordination to feed your brain, this section of the book will get you doing some fun eye-hand exercises and more. Yes, you will learn to juggle like the guys in the circus. However, we juggle balls, not chainsaws or fire…risk vs. reward.

I always did marvel at circus jugglers. The best I've seen can balance on almost anything, while having several balls (or whatever they use) in the air at once. They have mastered tapping into multiple systems and keeping them flowing. This is the epitome of the flow state ATHLETICISM is looking to achieve for athletes. I highlight juggling, but there are numerous Whole Brain exercises in our program. We do them all with the same intent of developing brain plasticity and tapping into the ultimate brain wave state.

I combine the three pillars of Awareness, Whole Body, and Whole Brain because you need every aspect of them to elevate your performance. I have met many athletes who are completely ambidextrous and could not compete under competition, playing at the pro level, because they needed the flow of this entire program. The body exercises simply help the brain develop faster improving vascular health in protecting and nurturing brain tissue, while challenging new connections. One of the main differences of ATHLETICISM Whole Body Whole Brain development is that we work unilaterally and bilaterally, synchronizing both sides of the body and both hemispheres of the brain equally and together, connecting them to the rest of the body. It is not only body fitness, but also brain fitness. Your eyes and ears carry some of the most primal reflexes and should be worked on along with all the other cranial nerves.

We stack the brain exercises with body exercises, challenging the nervous system at a deeper level. This multi-tier, integration approach stimulates the brain in new, challenging ways, allowing it to adapt and grow through brain plasticity. These types of exercises are rarely the focus for performance. I hope to change that. These exercises are addicting and never get old.

When individuals run, skip, bound, shuffle, and change directions in semicircles or do figure 8 movements, it works the brain in unbelievable ways. When we add more eye-hand, eye-foot, reaction and ambidexterity exercises, like balancing on a BOSU ball on one leg while juggling and adding math equations, your serotonin levels elevate. This creates a frequency resonance that body thrives in. This takes your brain and body plasticity beyond to another dimension. The Whole Brain techniques include:

1. Eye-hand/foot development
2. Ambidexterity
3. Eye speed and recognition
4. Light therapy
5. Sound therapy
6. Sensory nerve and motor nerve stimulation
7. Reaction development
8. Visualization
9. Focus and retention
10. Peripheral vision
11. Optikinetics
12. 6th sense intuition

Again, we integrate these or stack them in our sessions. Serotonin is an important chemical and neurotransmitter reward. It regulates function, mood, behavior, digestion, sleep, memory, sex drive, and appetite. Dopamine is another important neurotransmitter talking to the nerve cells with a long-term reward behavior. These are the stimuli to reward your new plasticity. Workouts that release these lead to another level of performance.

Once you start doing these exercises with some success, you will want to add what I call Athleticism Neuro Stacking development. This means stacking the exercises so that multiple systems of your body are working, integrated, and stressed appropriately, at the same time. This Athleticism

Neuro Stacking turns all systems 'On' from a mental, physical, and physiological standpoint engaging billions of neurons.

In our first Awareness pillar, we briefly mentioned that brain wave entrainment allows us to tap into a higher brain wave state. There are 4 main brain wave states to address:

1. Beta = wide awake and active
2. Alpha = calm and focused
3. Theta = creative and deeply meditative
4. Delta = low wave, deep, dreamless, and restorative sleep

Beta frequencies range from 12 Hertz to 40 Hertz (Hz) or cycles per second. Low or moderate beta amplitude connects to our state of alertness, thinking, and physical function. High amplitude is a fast beta, showing anxiety, discomfort, stress, and fight or flight state. Staying in this state will drain physical and emotional energy.

Alpha frequencies are found between 8 Hz to 13 Hz. This is when you are in more of a relaxed state with external focus. The higher alpha state represents a mindfulness state of relaxed and effortless alertness. The lower alpha state is more of a meditative state connecting with the subconscious mind. The alpha state is where peak performance and accelerated learning occurs. Mental rejuvenation from a peaceful nature walk will bring you to this level.

Theta brain frequencies range from about 3 Hz to 8 Hz. We find this state as we are just about to fall asleep during the REM sleep. This is where we can create vivid imagery before we wake to create our future. The Qi masters will find this in the deep meditative state. I use Dr. Schwartz's VIBE for sound and frequency healing. The Cell Cleanser mode will get you in a deep Theta state while detoxing and ridding inflammation. I also stack the treatment with Campo Beauty's Love essential oil, light therapy, and our Grounding Bags. It's the greatest full body immersive experience ever. When you connect to these low brain wave states on a regular basis, you will have better success entering the theta zone for performance and recovery. This is where we find heightened creativity.

Delta frequencies range from about 1 Hz to 3 Hz. This is where deep physical and mental regeneration occurs. Growth hormones are released during this dreamless deep sleep state during the natural sleep cycle. We want to maximize this state.

Optimizing all your brain waves, specifically your alpha state, will heighten your intuition, 6th sense, and extrasensory perception (ESP). In sports, when you can intuitively tap into the energy of your opponent, you will know exactly what he or she will do next. Some say they get lucky and guess right, but it is a lot deeper than that. You actually intuitively know exactly their next move. They may have a slight tell, are linearly trained to favor their go-to direction, or you just instinctively know their next move and are feeling their energy. All of those come from having a deeper level of intuition.

We connect into these desired levels through your heart by increasing your heart rate variability (HRV). This HRV connection is between your heart, brain, and nervous system. Our goal is to optimize brain wave levels and their consistency of rhythmic brain waves, thus promoting growth of neurotransmitters. HeartMath is a fantastic way to quantify where you are in the process. They have developed an app called Inner Balance. You plug a pulse reader into your phone and clip it to your ear lobe. It uses a math formula to convert your pulse to a heart rate variability. This heart coherence developed transfers into the flow state for performance.

If you are living in the frontal cortex of your head and thinking too much, your rhythm of variability will be low (score a 1). When you are leading with your heart, by emitting love and gratitude, your HRV will move upward toward scoring a 6. When you focus on breathing and your heart is full of love, this takes you into the parasympathetic mode, allowing your body to heal and flow. Plus, your HRV is directly correlated with your alpha levels. Basically, any exercise that makes you focus and stay in the moment and connected to your heart is beneficial. The trick is to maintain this consistently over extended periods of time and during competition. This will also raise your intuition. You will intuitively sense the next move, and you'll sense when something is right or not. This is one of the highest levels to develop. This requires raising all your frequencies to the optimal level, honing in on your craft, and sensing the energy of the competitor. You will flow effortlessly, and it is brilliant to feel and watch.

Make sure to get the HeartMath and MindSpa apps to help get your brain entrainment higher by learning how to meditate. Both our Whole Brain exercises and those two devices complement each other. The HeartMath will quantify everything and digitally let you know how you are progressing through their Inner Balance app. It is so cool to be able to feel it, see the results in your sport or endeavors, but it is awesome to quantify it as well.

You can walk up to anyone and test your level compared to his or hers. Most will likely start at a 1, unless they do lots of Qi Gong, meditation, or they know how to connect to the pineal gland when breathing. What a powerful tool to display how present and connected you are to your heart. This is yet another way to raise your consciousness and performance.

The MindSpa uses light and binaural beats to achieve your desired levels. Flickering light diodes reach the optic nerves coupled with sound. The strobes of light can alter your frequency following response now, called brain entrainment. These tools can passively get you in your target state as your brain follows suit. Add breathing and visualization to them for even better and faster results.

Finding these alpha states is important for everyone throughout the day, not just athletes competing. Every second of every thought counts to keep you in a higher state. When your muscles are more relaxed, you will expend less energy, and avoid a tight and stiff neck or other body parts. When the digestion system is relaxed, it flows better, and you will have stronger immunity. The big part is when you are in more of a meditative state, you will see an increase of blood carrying oxygen to the brain, leading to better decision making and clarity. You will also find an increase in serotonin. Consistent praying, going to church and praying with others, and maintaining a spiritual connection will drive this heightened level of consciousness.

When you don't have the assistance of these products, it may take years to find your optimal alpha state from meditation. Our ATHLETICISM Whole Brain program is designed to get you there a lot quicker with specific, fun exercises.

Ideally, it is best to start off with your cranial nerves firing on all cylinders. When we optimize the nerves through Athleticism Neuro Stacking, the body will come alive. In my practice, to expedite brain plasticity, I watch, correct, and treat my athletes when they are doing our ambidexterity exercises. I do not know many experts who work on nerve health with athletes, especially when athletes are doing other exercises. Most of the neuro doctors are doing incredible work on sick people or people who had massive accidents.

These ambidexterity exercises can be done any time of day. You can't do them too often. Your body will intuitively tell you when to move to the next exercise. This is not weight training where there are a specific number of sets and reps to do. You just play with our exercises. When you are stuck inside due to bad weather or fatigued on a body recovery day, it is the perfect way to make gains. Do them in between sets at the gym to keep your mind sharp. Practice at work. The exercises will boost your energy and get the creative juices flowing. Like the sports teams, you will develop a lot of fun, team synergy, especially in the corporate world. We will start with eye-hand exercises, the foundation for Whole Brain development. Below are multiple games, exercises, ideas, and activities that will keep you busy mastering them for the next two decades and beyond.

Cup Stacking.

I was hired by coach Dan Glenn, the legendary girls' varsity volleyball coach at Newport Harbor High School in Newport Beach, California. This is a volleyball mecca. He had a special team of girls. I was their speed, jump, and performance coach for the season. Each week, I worked with them twice a week into playoffs. Through developing their ATHLETICISM Whole Body Whole Brain, they won CIF and went on to play for a state title.

Coaches worry about whether their players are getting ahead of themselves before big games. My role is to prepare players for major competition. So, how do you prepare for the big game?

I was headed to Spain to work with Jordy Smith and the O'Neill surf team for their pro contest at Mundaka, so I wouldn't be there for Newport Harbor's state final pre-game warm-up. This meant that our last practice would set the tone. To get these girls in the flow, I pulled out my Speed Stacks.

The sport of cup stacking started in Oceanside, California, by Wayne Godinet out of the Boys and Girls Club. Bob Fox fell in love with the concept and brought a new line of cups to the market. He makes the fastest cups, called Speed Stacks. You must stack 12 cups in proper sequences. Wayne brought us some of the first cups ever made in the late 1990s. Bob elevated this sport globally. My fastest time was 11 seconds. If I dropped 1 more second off my time, I could have competed internationally. I got into this sport from working with my clients. We had and continue to have numerous epic battles. I use it as a mind and ambidexterity development tool. My hands got faster than ever through cup stacking. It's you against the clock, gravity, and your own coordination.

Preparing for the competition at Newport Harbor, I broke the girls into groups and had cup stacking races. We had one of the most exciting and fun sessions ever. I raised the intensity past their threshold and past the intensity they would see on their big game day. We had everyone involved and cheering. It really broke any tension in the air. They went into the state finals relaxed with the softest, quickest hands and went on to win state with ease!

Soft, quick hands, relaxed concentration, dexterity, ambidexterity, reflexes, performing under a timed, pressure situation, having external noise to cause even more distractions to improve your focus, adding a specific sequence to do in a set order using both hands equally…all this and more shows the power of cup stacking and Whole Body Whole Brain development.

Whole Brain development is for improving performance and preventing future brain challenges. All the brain memory challenges as we age can be delayed or avoided by keeping your brain sharp. We want to do more than just sitting and reading or doing puzzles to keep the brain firing on all cylinders. The aging slowdown of the brain happens over years. The Whole Brain connections can occur instantly. Doing these types of Whole Brain exercises may be the best for slowing down the aging process. Stacking cups would be ideal for elderly people, too.

Challenge the body appropriately, reduce inflammation, and develop more pathways from your brain to your body. It is not all about taking the latest supplement to develop these connections. It is about stressing the coordination of your body to achieve a Whole Body Whole Brain response. This is a simple term called adaptation. Our body loves to adapt when it is stressed appropriately. You will see the flow of your sport and other aspects of your life improve. Your energy, creativity, and clarity will increase. You will overall be in a happier mood with a bounce to your step.

Juggling.

Juggling is the essence of being a Whole Brain performer. Juggling is by far one of my favorite exercises to develop the Whole Body Whole Brain. It embodies the figure 8, rhythm, eye-hand coordination, dexterity, and processing systems. When someone is learning how to juggle, you can see their brain ticking. They know what they want to do, but the brain and their existing coordination fight it. How long will it take to learn how to juggle? Well, everyone is different and starts at different levels. The more you do it, the faster you will learn. Teaching someone to juggle is the best. You can see the brain ticking. The brain knows what to do, but the hands fight it. This newfound, Whole Brain exercise will allow you to play exceptionally better than before.

The simplest form of juggling is by using 3 balls. Start with 2 balls in one hand and 1 in the other. Starting with the hand that has 2 balls, lead with the outside ball. You toss each ball up to the other hand, one at a time. This creates the infinite figure 8. When someone is right (or one-side) dominant, they may have difficulty learning how to juggle. They will often pass the ball to the other hand instead of tossing it up to the other hand. Balls will get stuck in their hand, meaning they have a hard time tossing it up to the other hand and letting go of it. This just shows us that their brain is linearly developed and we can see it attempting to harness more plasticity.

It is similar to the "pat your head and rub your belly" exercise. The concept is easy to grasp, but since the brain has been linearly trained, the task is difficult to complete, as so many may rarely train to be a Whole Body Whole Brain performer.

When you learn the basic figure 8 juggling with 3 balls, you can branch out in endless ways to juggle from there. Train your peripheral vision by juggling and looking straight ahead, not at the individual balls. You can do that same basic figure 8 motion off the ground or wall. You can just get loose and have fun adding to your routine. I like to Neuro Stack, so we juggle while on a BOSU ball (standing on both legs, then only one leg) while you are adding math equations. Keep stacking exercises and being creative. Use different sizes and weighted balls and add more balls. Yes, it is the infinite flow taking you into the infinite mindset.

Want to learn how to juggle 4 balls? Start with 2 balls in one hand. Toss 1 up, then the next, in a circular flow. Once you get that flow in one hand, learn how to do the same thing in the other hand. Once you learn how to juggle 2 balls in the left hand, then 2 balls in the right hand, you can have a total of 4 balls (2 in each hand) and toss them up at the same time. The next progression is to alternate the timing of the start of the tosses in each hand. Make sure to keep the 2 balls in the circular flow in the same hand. When you get really good, you can pass the balls up and over to the other hand. This will develop those superhuman ambidexterity, processing skills you have been searching for.

Washers/Poker Chips.

Another of our go-to ambidexterity exercises is to put a poker chip, washer, or quarter on the top of your hand, with the palm facing down. You quickly raise your hand up, tossing the chip in the air. Then, swipe down to catch them, one at a time, keeping the palms facing down. We start with one hand, then the other, then both.

Next, we start to line the chips up your hand/arm, catching the one closest to you first. Start with 2 chips lined up the length of your arm. There are 2 distinctly different strokes when catching 1 chip at a time, with your palm facing away and down.

Then add a third, catching each chip with distinctly different strokes, one at a time. You must have soft, quick hands, dexterity, and sharp eye-hand coordination to catch each one. Get good at using both hands.

Next, we put 1 chip on each hand, tossing them up and catching them at the same time. We can keep adding chips. You can also alternate hands, catching the chip on the opposite hand, with the opposite hand. Make sure to toss them straight up and reach across.

Keep alternating chips as you add them. This looks like 2 chips on one hand and 1 on the other, alternating and catching the chips with the opposite hand. Let's start with 2 on the right hand and 1 on the left. You raise your arms, tossing them up at the same time. The left hand catches the one that is closest to you on the right hand. Then, the right hand catches the one that is on the left, and finish with the left hand catching the third chip.

Next, do the same alternating pattern starting with 2 chips on the left hand and 1 on the right. Then, build up to 2 on each hand and keep adding chips. See how fast you can get.

Speed, dexterity, eye-hand development, performing under pressure, staying in the moment, are all learned traits with this exercise. The Whole Body and Whole Brain is working and integrating when exercising ambidexterity. You must be so focused to throw 2, 3, or more up in the air and selectively catch 1 at a time. This is where all your breathing exercises come into play. You must slow it down and stay in the moment, even though it is all happening so fast. The hands are light, quick, and nimble. The eyes are mapping out the route (visualizing) before you start, then executing 1 at a time. These are the ways to make significant gains in becoming ambidextrous. You are rewiring your brain, creating more pathways from your brain to your body and the end points of your hands. This integration with progression will harness your inner genius faster than just reading books all day.

Dexterity Strength.

Not enough people develop coordination, flexibility, and strength in their hands and fingers. Of course, we do and now you will learn as well. There is so much potential in developing dexterity properly. Stretching and strengthening each finger and joint will provide tremendous coordination. Being able to use each joint effectively, having them long and stable will directly transfer into fewer errors and a better performance. Your head will feel new. In my clinic, I have an entire stretching and stability program for the hands. In this book, I will teach you our dexterity program to develop more coordination and ambidexterity in your hands.

Have you ever used 2 stress balls and circularly rotated them in your hand to reduce stress? We take that concept and use 2 pool balls. They are a bit larger, heavier, and the ideal weight to challenge the dexterity of your fingers.

Start with 2 pool balls in your dominant hand. Rotate them to your right or clockwise, then left or counterclockwise. Now, rotate them each direction without them separating from each other. The balls should not click apart. Next, rotate them each direction without them touching each other. Switch hands and repeat. Once you can do it in each hand individually, add 2 more balls, so you have 2 balls in each hand working at the same time. Go through this entire system together at the same time. Each hand going each direction, both the same direction at the same time, and the opposite direction at the same time.

When you get good at this, you can even add a third ball. Then add a fourth ball, literally on top of the three balls. There is no telling how good you can get. Each finger will develop more strength and coordination. You will soon learn to coordinate all fingers and both hands at the same time. When you first start to do 2 balls in one hand, you will find that it is easier for 1 of your hands to go a certain direction. These are the exact pathways we are opening up. The more you practice, the more dexterity you will develop in your hands. More dexterity in both hands transfers into greater performance and fewer, unforced errors.

One of my go-to finger strengthening exercises is to use a flat tennis ball or a dense foam ball, pinching it with each finger and your thumb individually, then collectively. The former Strength & Conditioning Coach/Athletic Trainer of the San Diego Padres, Bill Henry, invited me to work with the team. As I was going through the hand stretches and strengthening exercise, I handed out tennis balls to every player for strengthening exercises and juggling. One of the guys in the back was a pitcher who had worked with Aaron Mattes for years previously. He could crush the tennis ball with his pinky and thumb. It is absolutely incredible to have that strength in your pinky. I joked saying the ball was extra flat, but I validated that his skill was incredible! I hadn't seen many get strength to that extent. Every finger is so important for a pitcher to have maximal strength and dexterity.

A water polo ball is the perfect size and grip texture for most to train grip strength. I will palm it and lift my entire arm up, keeping the palm facing down. On every up movement, I let go of the ball and re-catch or palm it. I repeat this as many times as I can. The fingers get so strong doing this exercise.

Chapter 12: Eye Speed & Reaction Development.

Exercises to strengthen the eye muscles are one of the most missed elements of performance. Not many understand that you can actually do exercises that strengthen the muscles in each eye, to improve the fine motor skills of both eyes. In my clinic, I do the eye exercises and incorporate the nerve work to fire the muscles in the eyes. Light therapy has been an incredible part of my practice. Just to clarify, no, I do not shine light in the eyes. If an individual is not having proper eye recognition in sport, school, or work, this type of work will immediately change it. The sensory nerve health may be some of the most important work. When those major nerves are maximized, the entire body is upregulated.

We use eye exercises that allow you to strengthen the nondominant eye. This will help improve your vision. I lock my eyes in before I play any sport, just as I teach to stabilize the joints and muscles. The results are tangible as you will play with incredible accuracy. A cross-eyed method is one go-to exercise. This uses two identical pictures, adjacent to each other, and you do a cross-eyed method to create a third equal one in the middle. The farther apart the two same pictures are, the harder it will be to create the third equal one.

There are great online sites for memory and eye exercises. Visualization, or what we call imagery exercises, is another major complement to eye development. When you can create a detailed visual image of yourself performing, coupled with all the colors, smells, sounds, tastes, and more, it will help the actual performance and improve your performance when it is live. When you have seen what is coming, your body responds. In addition to the other ambidexterity exercises, this is one simple exercise you can do anywhere.

Go to a bead store and get about 7 large beads and about a 50" string. Put the beads on the string and tie knots at each end. Space the beads out equally on the string by having a friend hold one end of the string while you hold the other. Put the string up to the tip of your noses.

Look at each bead, one at a time, starting with the one closest to you. Using this cross-eyed method, you should see two strings going into the center of the bead. Make sure you can see both strings and quickly get them to enter the center of the bead. Progress the eyes to the next bead, going all the way to the end and back. Next, start skipping beads and being creative about bouncing from bead to bead, teaching your eyes to pick up the next bead as quickly as possible.

If one line of the string is fainter than the other, it is the opposite eye that needs more work. This is called the cross-eyed method of eye development. The more you practice, the quicker you will pick up each bead. Plus, you can increase the string to about 12 feet and strengthen the range of your eyes.

Having played lots of sports, I would always hear the coach say, "Keep your eye on the ball!" It is to this day the best, most underrated tip that anyone could give. So many people have a hard time tracking the ball all the way into their hands, glove, racquet, club, bat, or whatever your sport requires. Most will close their eyes before they catch or hit the ball. Keeping your eye on the ball also means to watch the seams, color, writing, or shadow of the ball. What is the last part of the ball you saw? Watch the ball all the way into the hands or whatever object the ball is supposed to meet. Practice catching a ball behind where you would normally make contact. This will teach you to track in an even bigger range of motion. So, when you go back to hitting, it is easy to follow the ball all the way into the bat.

Another drill I like to do with baseball and softball players is to teach them to see and hit small objects. When athletes can take a thin stick and hit a small bean, it develops their eyes, timing, focus, and fine motor skills.

I have used a Swift Stick for years. We get bags of beans and soft toss them to the hitter. We start with the hitters making contact when on the ground. Then, we will have them stand on a Figure 8 Board or BOSU ball when hitting. This ties into our Neuro Stacking concept. What a great exercise to build the hitter's confidence. If they can hit a tiny little bean with a skinny stick on a balance product, they sure can hit a big baseball or softball.

The founder of the BOSU ball, David Weck, is quite an inventor. He has invented several products in addition to his famous BOSU ball. He invented a reaction trainer called the BOSU Bola Reactionary Trainer that is amazing for developing ambidexterity, eye speed, and reflexes. It is no longer in production, but I still have several. They are 2 foam balls, each the size of a tennis ball, with a 16" bungee cord connecting the balls. I have had clients make their own out of a bungee cord and 2 tennis balls. There are endless exercises with this product.

When you are doing Whole Brain development, your eyes are key. The more developed your fine motor and spatial skills are, the better you will play. We use an eye poster developed by the late Dr. Bill Harrison. It has balls numbered 1 to 50, in a mixed order. We tie in movement with eye speed and recognition exercises for endless exercises.

We have athletes point with their right hand on the odd numbers and left hand on the even numbers. They are racing another person while standing on a BOSU ball. If someone falls off, they have to back up 5 numbers. This timed, pressure race, integrating balance and hand movements, is excellent for developing the Whole Brain and learning how to perform under timed, pressure situations. To raise the stakes and make yourself concentrate even more, you can have a few people distracting you and talking to you while concentrating. It is too fun and really challenging. That eye chart is an integral part of our Whole Brain development program.

In addition to the nerve restoration with light therapy, I use some of Montak Chia's Qi Gong exercises to soothe and heal the eyes. First, put your hands in front of your eyes just a few inches away. Close your eyes and synchronize your hands and eyes moving right to left 16 times, then in circles, both directions, 16 times. Next, place your hands on the eyes and send them Qi. Lastly, with your eyes closed, rub your eyeball in small circles all around it. Also rub the back of the head, opposite of the eyes. Give your eyes Infinite Love & Gratitude. These are the restorative eye exercises.

ATHLETICISM

Chapter 13: Games & Ambidexterity Exercises.

Let's dive into more fundamental ambidexterity exercises.

Throwing & Hitting: When throwing a ball, connect to the concept of opposite and equal while using a figure 8 movement system. This allows the power to come from your core without any opposing friction on the throwing arm. This enforces the figure 8, opposite and equal, throwing movement where the dog (hips), wags the tail (the arm). Opposite arm, opposite leg throwing maintains the proper cross-crawl energy. Put it all together, initiating from the core, and you will have a coordinated, accurate, and powerful throw.

Practicing with the non-dominant hand will feel very awkward at first. The more you throw with it, the easier it gets. Maintaining consistency with this is key. Doing it once or twice will not have the lasting effects we are looking for. I am talking about doing these throwing games over the years. My daughter is now 12, and we still use both sides when we play. In fact, she now initiates throwing and hitting with the opposite hand because she knows it gives her an edge. She still has a dominant right hand, no question. But her coordination on the opposite hand is better than most people's dominant side. She played water polo for the first time and can pass, catch, and throw with both hands. We have epic battles playing ping-pong or table tennis with both hands. It is so fun!

The same holds true for swinging a bat, club, or tennis racquet with both hands. The great doctors, like Tim Brown, DC, (founder of IntelliSkin.net) saw so many imbalances in his athletes from posture and overuse on one side. Years ago, he gave clinical treatment protocols for the athletes to balance out their muscles by swinging opposite handed. That is why we collaborate and get along so well today. Prior to our meeting, we both recognized that Whole Body Whole Brain ambidexterity development separates the pack in performance and injury prevention. We take that out-of-the-box approach to everything we do. Dr. Brown's younger brother, Bill Brown, DC, also emphasizes this approach when doing performance work with his athletes. The guys who do this get incredible results.

·····································

Writing is something that nearly everyone does every day. For kids, have them write their name on a paper with their opposite hand. For adults, sign your name at the checkout counter with your opposite hand. It doesn't have to be perfect. The intent is simply to use your other hand. Keep it short and unlock those pathways.

For those who like to draw, practice with your opposite hand. Switching from right to left hand may smear your work and get ink all over your hand, but it will give you a different perspective on drawing.

Coloring with the opposite hand is one of my favorites, especially now that I have a child. Every restaurant we go to has a kid's menu to color. Grab an extra one and fill it out with crayons. Staying in the lines can be quite challenging, especially for the adults.

···

You knew this was on the list. Kick with both feet. I was the assistant coach for my daughter's AYSO a few seasons back. We went from a 0-3 start to the finals by teaching the kids how to actually kick a ball. Very few coaches focus on learning the fundamentals of kicking. It was incredible to see the improvements. When we got the kids using both feet, we ended up dramatically improving our play.

When kicking a soccer ball with your right foot, step next to the ball with the left, and then kick the ball with the right. Do the same on the other side. The planted foot should point directly toward where you are kicking the ball. Kick with the laces toward the instep that are the metatarsal, cuneiform, and navicular bones. Point the toe down (not flexed). Make sure you follow through the ball and drive the knee up to the chest. Lean forward and keep the eyes open, watching the foot hit the ball. Leaning back on contact will lift the ball over the goal. Those few tips should get you started.

....

Many of the X-Games sports and others, including skiing, snowboarding, surfing, skateboarding and figure skating, are all so fun to watch now because the athletes spin during their flip. The parkour crew has made everyone step up their game. Trampoline houses are everywhere, so you can practice rotational flips and land in a foam pit without a worry. This type of athletic development will facilitate more spatial awareness.

....

One of the things my daughter did the most from age 4 to 8 was cartwheels. She must have done at least 100 per day. One day, we were at my daughter's dance class and there was a gymnast doing flawless cartwheels repeatedly. I, of course, had her face the same direction and do a cartwheel to the right. Then to the left. She wanted to turn so badly to face the other direction. Here is someone who had done flawless cartwheels for years and never thought to go back the other direction. It took her about 10 minutes to figure it out. We could see her brain plasticity working throughout the process. Practice keeping the arms slightly bent so they don't become hyper mobile. If a joint is too mobile, it opens for future injuries. Joints need to be pliable but stable. I noticed that in her as well.

....

Monkey bars are back in style, thanks to crossfit, muscle ups, and American Ninja Warrior with their climbing moves. The pull-up is one of the most functional exercise for the back. Before you can actually pull yourself up, just hanging from the bar will get you started. When swinging from bar to bar, make sure to lead with each hand. This will balance out the strength and coordination on both sides.

Simulation rock climbing gyms are ideal places to learn to climb. You can take your cross-crawl, bear crawl patterns to the wall. They have automatic belays that, once clipped in, keep you safe from falling. They have timers to see how efficiently you can climb the wall. Mapping out the first few steps before you start will improve your time. So, make sure there is a foot and handhold for the first and second steps. This will save at least several seconds off the time for most people. This is also a great exercise to keep you in a parasympathetic mode.

·································

There are numerous applications for ambidexterity work even when you aren't really doing much. Crossing legs and arms opposite of your default is a perfect example. It feels awkward to have the arms switched. If you are married, you can show your ring off easier with the fingers resting on the outside of the arm.

You can take this same concept to sports activities. Even when diving in the water, switch which hands are on top. Or pushing off the wall when swimming and doing a flip turn, flip to the left and right. Did someone say, "Endless?"

Here is something we do every day…stepping onto a curb or a step. Do you always lead with the same leg? Step up stairs with the left leg first, then lead with the right leg first. The goal is to make the brain realize that there is no difference as to which leg steps first. We do this same development in our foam barrier drills.

Play the bongos with both hands. Drummers are ambidextrous. Just using the other hand is the starting point. Bang that drum more times with the non-dominant hand. It's a fun and easy way to do Whole Brain development.

Dribble a basketball with both hands. As you improve, dribble 2 basketballs at the same time, 1 with each hand. Alternate dribbling in different directions. Shoot with both hands, of course. Repetition is key. Have a shooting contest with a friend. I can't tell you, still to this day, how many elite performers do not understand the concept of using both sides of their body.

I was shooting baskets at the gym at the same time as a collegiate D1 basketball player who just graduated. He will be playing professionally in Asia soon. Before I took a break, he saw me working on athletes and asked what I do. I gave him a brief description of our performance program working on nerves, whole body, and whole brain. I noticed he was a linearly trained and needed to do some ambidexterity work to take his game to the next level. I mentioned that an equal majority of my warm-up shots are done with my non-dominant hand. He said, "Interesting," and proceeded to shoot with his right hand only. Every basketball player should be lethal with both hands from the free throw line in. Until he becomes a Whole Brain Whole Body performer, he will most likely stay in Asia and not make the NBA. All I know is that if I were remotely close to 7 feet tall, I would have played in the NBA from this type of Whole Brain development.

....

Survival instincts are considered primal reflexes of the body. Fight, freeze, or flee are reflexes most of us have experienced in one form or another. Since our nerve health determines our overall health, it is so important to get back to connecting with our survival instincts. Not necessarily getting scared out of your pants, but more so feeling the fight instinct to keep you alive and thriving. To thrive we need to get back to the roots of developing those instincts. Boxing, shadow boxing, running, and kicking are some of my favorites as well. I will often shadow box in the water. I can get faster muscle twitch to fire on both sides of my body and get my heart rate up quickly.

....

Connecting the core to cross-crawl patterns in different planes is important. Exercises like a cross-crawl plank will connect cross patterns while engaging the core with opposite hand or elbow and foot supporting the body. Once in push-up position, raise the opposite arm and leg at the same time. Bear crawls are fun, ambidextrous exercises that also develop coordination and strength in a different plane. If you want a good core workout, start on the stomach and go into a plank position. Then do bear crawls forward, backward, and side to side, lifting the opposite hand and leg at the exact same moment. Gymnastics offers amazing strength development in this plane, which is also great for jujitsu and breakdancing.

....

When you begin to learn how to snowboard, you'll be asked which foot you want as your front foot. Are you regular or goofy footed? To figure out the answer, the common question is, "If you were to run and do a standing slide on ice or in your socks on a wood floor, which foot would you lead with?" Most right-handed individuals have their right foot back. They call the ones with the left foot back, goofy footers. Either way, you know to learn both ways to tap into your Whole Body Whole Brain. Starting on a razor scooter is the easiest to teach switch stance because you can hold on to the handle. I teach both regular and goofy skateboard, snowboard, and even surfing now. The tricks and turns are so dynamic now. Athletes should know how to seamlessly switch up their stance.

One of my favorite products for the new year is the B3 Bands. Dr. Mike DeBord has put together a special product. Athleticism.b3sciences.com has all the incredible studies on the growth factors, and you can purchase the bands. Blood flow restriction (BFR) has been too risky until now. The B3 Bands have airways so you are always getting oxygen. It is more like resistance than restriction. It is not a painful tourniquet. With less load, intensity, and duration, you can take your muscles into a deep burn. This will develop so much nitric oxide and vascular endothelial growth factor production of natural human growth hormones (HGH). The benefits are unlimited. You can heal injuries faster. Many will see their strength, speed, and power increase in just a few months. Doing 10-20 minute workouts three times per week will give you fantastic results. This is yet another way to make significant gains without heavy lifting and going into cortisol fatigue. Any time you can add subtle resistance to the body, it is designed to adapt. These bands will accelerate substantial gains at any level.

Conclusion: The Infinite Flow.

After spending decades studying the body and brain, I have learned performance comes down to how much of a Whole Body Whole Brain performer you are. Using this book as a road map, you can learn how you are designed and overachieve on your brain and body types and genetics. It is that awareness that will dictate the outcome of how you feel and perform. You will see things others don't. You will feel things others don't. You will have superior preparation. You will have more energy and a clearer mind. Your body will flow like never before. The energy of flowing in the moment will effortlessly go your way. This program will support you going to the highest level that you choose to go.

To see your own transformations occur, start to slowly incorporate this new level of awareness. I continue to learn what food my body thrives on, as it is an ever-changing process. I spent years learning to juggle like a pro and still practice it regularly. I spent years building my ATHLETICISM by doing our entire Whole Body Whole Brain ambidexterity program. It is a lifestyle, not a sip of a drink that you taste once and either like it or not. You actually have to work and be aware and creative about how you approach life and every activity that comes your way. I use the figure 8 in all my workouts. This lifestyle brings energy, awareness, health, and fun, yielding productivity and success. The path is there for you to take. You can choose how powerful you want to become.

When you burn fat as your primary fuel source, your body will transform. Purchase quality food and your life will reward you with sustained energy and vitality. Proper gut health will drive your energy and vitality, allowing you to fend off other stressors with ease. Plus, your cognitive decisions will be clearer than ever. Either you keep to the status quo, or you turn the page and heighten your awareness and health to a new level. I believe in the zest for life, learning, and growing.

To tie together this entire book there is no better suggestion than to use Cereset to help get your brain in sync. Cereset is a closed chain sound echo program that uses diodes to measure your brain wave activity and directly play music to get it back into sync. For those in need of assistance in taking their brain back to its primal state of being balanced, this is the program for you. They have franchises across the country. Balancing the right and left hemispheres of your brain leads to all the good sleep, health, and performance that I wrote in this book.

God gave us a third eye and a sixth sense of intuition. Developing optimal energy, speed, and performance through ATHLETICISM is my form of extrasensory perception or ESP. Learn how to breathe and listen to your body. Your body talks to you in so many ways. Let's make it as energetic, as fast, and as powerful as possible.

Last story…I have a client who had hip surgery. I now call him "one hip guy." Ok, another bad joke to end the book. He was an excellent athlete. About 10 years ago, his wife jumped in the pool and accidently landed on his hip. He attempted to stretch and shake off the injury. He never got an adjustment. Just feeling tighter on one side, he continued to use it and play hard. Progressively, his hip got worse to the point that he needed surgery. Looking back, a few chiropractic adjustments may have prevented him from having to go through a major hip replacement surgery. When there is metal on metal in a ball and socket joint, common in hip replacements, he would have to do heavy metal detoxes annually. This is the exact awareness we are talking about. Simple corrections can improve a lifestyle, quality of life, and avoid many of the future challenges, like a major surgery.

After reading this, you have the awareness and road map to go beyond. Start juggling, becoming an ATHLETICISM Whole Brain Whole Body performer, and get in the infinite flow.

You just learned the 3 pillars of performance:

1. Awareness
2. Whole Body Development
3. Whole Brain Development

It is now up to you to take your game to the next dimension.

Put these secrets, protocols, and methodologies to work to unlock the best version of you! Be happy, healthy, laugh, smile, giggle, and live life to the fullest. Expand with an abundance of infinite love, light, blessings, health, prosperity, laughter, and gratitude. Using our ATHLETICISM coordination programs, I invite and encourage you to have the most optimized and fulfilled life. Get outside. Take in, breathe, and connect with the energies of the earth, sun, and do what you love. Look into sound, light, and frequency healing. Please share this book and these methods with others. Thank you for your assiduous attention to your own welfare and taking this journey with me.

Gratitude.

When I write a book that covers the span of my entire life, I have a few thank-yous. The subject of this book would not be written if I hadn't met Dean Brittenham. Thank you, Dean, for being the biggest inspiration in my career. You provided me a direction that has filled my heart and soul with endless passion. Anyone who knows me refers to me as the ATHLETICISM guy. I could not be prouder. I am honored and privileged to share your work and be able to add to it. I thank God for allowing me to listen to my intuition and to step outside conventional thinking in learning about ATHLETICISM and how to facilitate in making athletes better.

This book would not have been completed if my editor, Heather Marsh, had not put her impressive editing skills to work. There are computer programs that edit books, but they will never touch the quality and passion of her work. As a health industry expert, Heather brought invaluable insight and wisdom beyond. There is no bigger praise that I can give anyone for being so exceptional at what they do. Thank you, Heather, for being such an incredible editor and friend. Thank you for allowing me to work on you and your kids to actually see and experience all that I have written. Thank you for believing in me and facilitating in sharing my work with the masses. Thank you for all you did to make my book come to life. Infinite love and gratitude.

In no particular order, I want to thank every name that I mentioned in this book and give some special gratitude. You all have touched my life in a positive way, and I am grateful. As Kent Ewing taught me, I want to thank all my previous clients as they took part in teaching me.

Jess, you nailed the cover, as always. You are my inspiration, you are my love, you are my everything. Thank you for bringing out the best in me. Thank you for being so patient with me and always having my back. My love and respect for you is so strong. You are the most talented, supporting, giant hearted wife and Mom on the planet. Your creative genius is unmatched in every way. I am so proud of all your accomplishments. Campo Beauty is taking the clean beauty market to an entirely new level. I love you!! 143, Full Power!

Lauren, thank you for being you and always putting a smile on my face. You have the biggest, most beautiful heart, soul, and spirit, with gifts beyond. I am so proud of you. Every moment with you is my favorite part of the day. You bring light to the world that is brighter and more powerful than the sun. Let's keep having fun riding mountains, waves, and horses. You are always protected from above. I love you always!!

Mom and Dad, thank you for your unwavering love and support my entire life. Thank you for providing me with the education to be able to do what I do. It is a great honor to have you as family. You have always been so present in my life, and I am so grateful. Every foundation to be good, do good, and connect to God stems from your parenting. Thank you for being such powerful role models and guiding me to follow my dreams.

Graham, thanks for being an awesome brother. It was so much fun growing up with you as my Big Bro. You are the fun factor. Thanks for always being my biggest fan. You taught me to be the toughest guy possible.

Judi, thank you for all your energy, love, and support you have provided me and my entire family. You have filled our lives with smiles, fun, and a passion for horses. Your generosity and dedication to my family is incredible, and you are loved. Waves of love and gratitude.

Robb, to the giant hearted, generous, hospitality king. Thanks for keeping the male energy strong and all your warm and festive meals. You know how to dominate a BBQ, and I love our steak family meals. Con taught you well. love and light.

Chelsea, hey Sis! You bring the soothing pulse of warmth. Thanks for believing in me and seamlessly combining our families with big hugs. Lots of love.

Chloe & Chase, so fun seeing you shine in what you love. Keep bringing your brilliant talents to the world. Blessings and gratitude.

Ryan, proud of you for your awareness! It far surpasses the norm, and I am so excited to see how you continue to shine and follow your heart. Blessings and light.

Mike & Anthony, I appreciate you both and the fun you bring. Let's play some golf. Blessings and gratitude.

Paul, we have so much fun spending time with you. Thank you for your love, interest, and support in all our endeavors. Lauren adores you, Jess credits you for all, and I can't wait to do some organic and biodynamic farming with you. ;-)

AT & DOD, oh what fun...love and gratitude.

Thank you, Dr. Dreyer, for sharing offices with me for the past couple years. I could not have a better teacher and person by my side every day.

Stephen Stiteler, you saved my life and started me down this holistic path. Thank you for being such an amazing friend and healer.

Dr. Cohn, brother! Thank you for being such an incredible friend. It is a blast hosting our GoBeyondSummit.com together. The Cohn Health Institute is the best, and so are you and your wife, Dr. Christine. Your molecular hydrogen supplement, Recovery, is amazing. I know your sister, Linda Cohn, has broadcasted more Sports Centers than anyone, but you have helped more people than anyone. Can you say, Talented Beyond?!

Thank you to all the athletes, teams, corporations, and coaches that I have worked with and are currently working on ATHLETICISM. Facilitating making you the best allows me to share my gifts. For that, I am grateful.

Kent Ewing, what can I say? You are unbelievably incredible! Thank you for teaching me how to giggle and so much more. Love, light, blessings, and gratitude. Why not?!

Dr. Zach Bush, wow, what a legend! Thanks for being a true friend and making the biggest footprint (pun intended) on our world.

Thank you to all my healers and facilitators. Most are mentioned in the book, and the others…you know who you are.

Aaron Mattes, thank you for creating such an amazing stretching system. Your AIS system is a new lease on life for everyone.

Dr. Darren Weissman, this one is easy…*Infinite Love & Gratitude!*

A big thanks to USC. The Entrepreneur program taught me to do this on my own. The Exercise Science program taught me the basics. Thank you for the education.

Thanks, JBell, for being a SEAL and entrusting me to work on you and your son. Infinite thanks in writing the foreword to this book. Your heart and talents are beyond impressive.

Dr. Tim Brown, thanks for referring so many of your professional athletes to me and keeping me standing tall with your IntelliSkin. I love the saying, "Lead with your heart." That is the wisdom you instill in everyone's posture and body who wears your IntelliSkin.

Dr. John Pecora, thank you for all your help developing teams and supporting ATHLETICISM for so many years. You are such an impressive pro.

Dr. KFC, DAOM, skills beyond! Blessings and gratitude.

Jeremy Niednagel, thank you and your dad for bringing us brain typing. Thank you for your wisdom brain typing me and my family. God bless!

Barance Batos, you are the most exceptional sports massage therapist I've ever experienced. Thank you for getting those hard to reach places and getting me back on the basketball court.

Dr. Billy Brown, thanks for the friendship and amazing work. It is refreshing seeing you doing true performance work with incredible athletes, too.

Dr. David Karaba, thanks for your acupuncture, allergy elimination treatments, and getting my energy on point.

John Cook, thanks for years of fun and an incredible run. You are the Sportsman of the Year and of an entire career. Aloha!

You are the man, Fuerby! What an amazing friend…so aware and connected. Thanks for sharing so many AVP wins with me. You are the best 6'8" surfer I've seen. *Let's surf.*

Dr. Barre Lando & Mike Winner, thanks for creating such clean Alfa Vedic supplements and showing everyone that organic farming is the key to wellness and energy. You make my favorite supplements and are legendary in every way.

To Shane Kilcoyne, Johnny Drennen, and my Shibo Crew… ATHLETICISM 4 Life!

Joseph Gonzalez, thanks for the lifelong friendship and being the best ATHLETICISM ambassador and all your behind-the-scenes support with our GoBeyondSummit.com.

Dr. Dave Jensen, thanks for licensing ATHLETICISM and selling our Grounding Bags. Your friendship means everything. You are world class in every way and the person to see in Aspen. *Let's Ride!*

Lissa Trevino, thanks for bringing in ATHLETICISM to Ocean Physical Therapy.

Dr. Michael Gooing, thanks for getting to the root cause, helping me detox, and bringing my health back up to full strength. Brilliant!

Bill Henry, thanks for being such a pro…much respect!

Dr. Daniel Helm, you're awesome…blessings!

Dr. George Gonzalez, thank you for showing me the Light.

Dr. Charlie, your treatments are life savers…thank you!

To the O'Neill crew and Garth, so many fun times. Keep charging!

Kaleigh Gilchrist, you are pure gold and the best two-sport female athlete of our era. Water polo and surfing beyond. Fight on!

Peter Smith, your camps and Pepperdine team were some of my favorite times. Stoked you had such an impressive run in the Trojan Family. Thanks…fight on!

Dr. Rob Rettig, I know I'm not supposed to tell everyone what an incredible, inspirational doc you are, but too late. Thanks for making my Grounding Bags an integral part of your patients' *lives.*

Pedram Shojai, it was so fun connecting with you at the start of the movement.

John Iams, you are my Nobel Prize winner. PRRT is something every practitioner should know. Infinite gratitude.

Dr. Tom Bayne, thanks for your support and creating MegaSporeBiotic.

David Weck, I love the WeckMethod and all your inventions! Thank you for your work to evolve the industry. It is revolutionary.

Steve Cotter, thanks for bringing kettlebells into my world years ago.

Jerzy Gregorek, I knew nothing about O lifting until you taught me. Thank you for sharing your knowledge.

Dr. Ward Henry, thank you for teaching me your incredible manual nerve program. You are the best Jump Doc.

Dr. Toby Watkinson, you started all this nerve stability work! Thank you for being my go-to guy, especially when I was in SD. So excited to keep learning from you. Thanks for your continued support of my Grounding Bags.

lululemon, you make the best pants. Thanks for making my wife a lululemon Ambassador. All the managers, you rock!

Hoag, you have one of the most impressive teams and leadership I have ever seen. Thank you, Marcy and Robert, for believing in Jess, Campo, and for making us feel part of the family. We love integrating our approaches with your Hoag family.

Coach Steve Conti, thanks for being so open to ATHLETICISM with CDM Volleyball and my concussion treatments. Our surf sessions are my favorite.

Coach Glenn, fun run with your Newport Harbor teams and camps. Much gratitude.

Ron Jensen, thanks for being a great client, friend, and mentor. Your *Framework* books are amazing.

Dave Post, you are an incredible surf coach. Thanks for all the continued support. Look forward to surf trips ahead.

Eaglewoman, you gave me the most profound treatment of my life. Thank you for being a true shaman and helping me so much with your gifts.

Jason Hanck, you fine specimen. Thanks for spreading your Qi, wisdom, and pure love of life.

JB Green, thank you for allowing me to be part of your successful high school and collegiate football and volleyball careers. Fight on!

Paul McDonald, thanks for your continued support, allowing me to work with you and your sons, and for bringing awareness in athletes.

Jack Broudy, thanks for teaching me the figure 8 in sports.

Wake UP OC, Brad Axelrad, Steven E. Schmitt, thanks for facilitating in waking everyone up.

Troy Casey, AKA, The Certified Health Nut. It is so fun meeting people as authentic as you, who are making a significant impact on so many. Thank you for letting all know that I am not the only health nut out there. Blessings, gratitude, and liquid sunshine.

Tom Ritz, thanks for the lifelong friendship and support of ATHLETICISM. You have always had an incredible approach to performance.

Courtney Conlogue, all I can say is, you are the most aware, Whole Body Whole Brain performer I have had the pleasure to work with. WSL and the entire world, enjoy watching her shine and win! Let's paddle.

Ella Olson and all of Lauren's fenom friends, this book was written for you. I look forward to facilitating your athletic development, watching you turn pro, excel, and have lots of fun. There is no upper limit for you.

Dr. Calvin, it is refreshing to see such a young functional athlete and doctor doing everything recommended and taking care of oneself. Thank you for your solid treatments. You are the only doctor who stays with me and actually does workouts with over 100 pull-ups. Much respect.

Aaron, thanks for bringing frequency healing to the masses and being such a huge fan of our Grounding Bags. You are a wizard and Q360 Club is incredible.

Dr. Jack, thank you for being such a solid friend and introducing my Grounding Bags to NY.

Dr. Mary, so much gratitude for your treatments.

Kerri Schuh, you are pure ATHLETICISM as a pro athlete and artist. Thank you for the amazing illustrations in this book.

Rhonda, thank you for introducing me to Cereset and balancing my brain back to its primal state. It was the missing link for me. God bless!

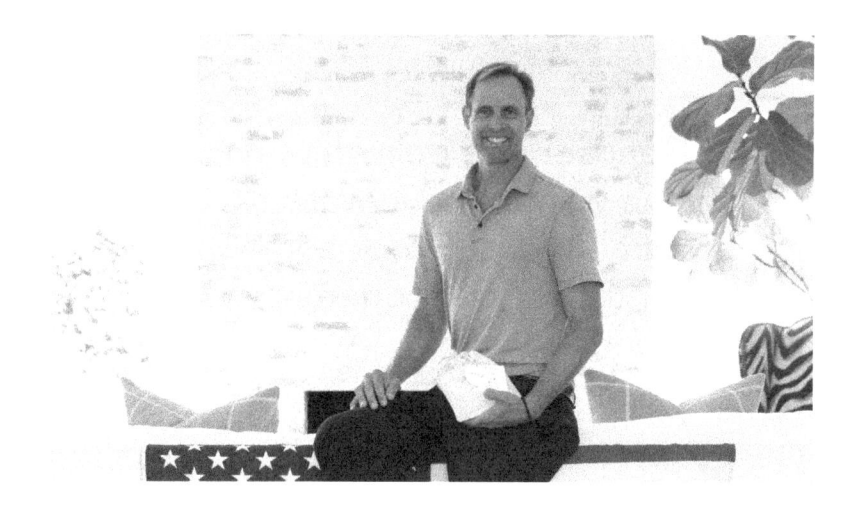

Leading the direction of human performance, Justin Frandson transcribes his journey and career of improving energy, speed, and performance. In 1994, after graduating from the University of Southern California (USC) Entrepreneur program and getting his EMT certification from UCLA, Justin had already awakened the health space being gluten free for several years. Once he met the legendary track and field coach, Dean Brittenham, ATHLETICISM started to take shape. It all began at the prestigious Scripps Clinic, in La Jolla, California, working with amateur and professional athletes in most major sports.

Justin expanded on what Dean developed, harnessing true performance through the most aware and creative approaches. The Whole Body exercises teach running, skipping, bounding like you've never seen with rhythms, coordinations in figure 8 patterns, and more. The Whole Brain approach covers everything from ambidexterity exercises, brain entrainment, to sensory nerve work. Justin dives deeply to provide tangible programs and protocols for your ultimate development, for any age.

Enjoy this fun read and storytelling about some of the greatest athletes from multiple sports. Many would call it a holistic approach. Justin would agree and add that it is an 'aware' approach. Justin is honored to share this proven program, providing you an easier, more seamless path to fulfilling your endeavors.

> Justin Frandson has delivered a must-read for anyone wanting to elevate their game to new dimensions. Finally someone has conveniently put it all together in this breakthrough system!
>
> Charlie Fagenholz,
> DC, PAK, Dip.H.Ir, QNCP
>
> Co-author of, *Autism Reimagined*

> Justin Frandson IS THE MAN! From a health perspective, both physically and philosophically, he stands in integrity where his mind, his heart, and his gut are aligned literally and figuratively! This is a must read for all.
>
> Troy Casey
> AKA, Certified Health Nut
>
> Author of, *#Ripped At 50*